I0541549

BEDSIDE

Nursing Stories

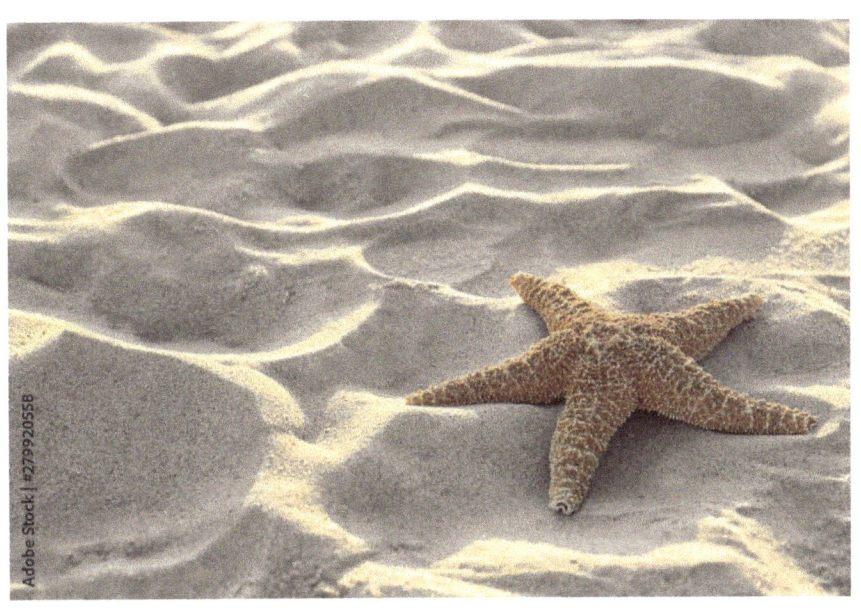

Adobe Stock | #279920558

Mary T. Russell EdD MSN

THE STARFISH STORY

One day a man was walking along the beach when he noticed a boy picking up and gently throwing things into the ocean.

Approaching the boy he asked: "Young man, what are you doing?"

The boy replied, "Throwing starfish back into the ocean. The surf is up and the tide is going out. If I don't throw them back, they'll die."

The man laughed to himself and said, "Do you realize there are miles of miles of beach and hundreds of starfish?" "You can't make any difference."

After listening politely, the boy bent down, picked up another starfish and threw it into the surf, then smiling at the man, he said; **"I made a difference to that one."**

— Loren Eiseley

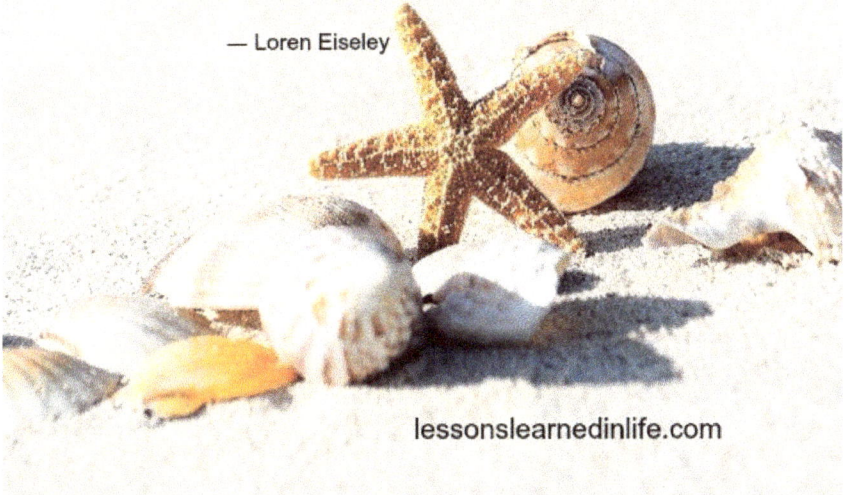

lessonslearnedinlife.com

Dedication

To past, present and future nurses who save lives and lifetimes, who give comfort and hope, make pain more bearable, and serve as angels to those in need of care.

Disclosure

The names of patients in the following stories have been changed for privacy.

Table of Contents

PROLOGUE

What is it that prompts the decision to become a nurse? What qualities constitute the "it" factor for such a career? My own opinion is that there may be many reasons. Personal experience of being the patient in the bed is one, perhaps taking care of a family member who is ill or injured, being a "helper" in life, intrigued by the mysteries of medicine, or maybe for some people, it is determining that you will always have a job anywhere you go as there will always be people who need care.

I have thought deeply about why I became a nurse and believe that such a life choice is more complex than any one incident. In my case, experiencing trauma early in my life and growing up in a large family was impactful. Health and safety public information and awareness was limited, especially when it came to understanding how our bodies work. Access to guidance was also restricted.

When I was in high school in the late 1960s, there were not many options for female careers. We were told that we had a choice of becoming a secretary, a nurse, a teacher, or getting married. Males had many more options. Today, it is still a choice to become a nurse, and gender is no longer a barrier.

Maybe it was always there- the need and decision to become a nurse. For me, it began in childhood experiencing what it was like to be a patient. I felt vulnerable and scared and did not understand the language being spoken in an unfamiliar place that was full of scary equipment and unknown procedures. I had to trust those who cared for me.

I remember searching our local small library for books about nursing and was disappointed. I craved learning more about the field of healthcare and reading real stories, not dramatized fiction. I have learned that every nurse has stories, and we are inherently storytellers as we report to colleagues to continue to care for our patients.

My career has now spanned 48 years and spanned a journey within critical care units, burn units, emergency departments, and public health. I mostly worked night shifts as that gave me more flexibility to raise children and to be able to get involved in activities aligned with my interest in injury prevention and disaster preparedness. In the endless stream of patients, I have cared for over the years, there are some that are never forgotten. This book offers a glimpse into the real world of bedside nursing, as seen through my own experience over time.

PART ONE
My Personal Journey toward a Career Decision

The First Stages of a Master Plan. 1953-1960

My parents waited until my 13th birthday to tell me about my early story. I was born in Mount Vernon, New York, on December 26, 1953, as the second of nine children in my family. Apparently, when I was six weeks old, my mom noticed that I did not blink when her hand went near my eyes while bottle-feeding me. Our pediatrician confirmed this finding and referred my parents to take me to an Eye Specialty Hospital in New York City, Columbia Eye & Ear.

I was admitted there and underwent some type of procedure under general anesthesia. My parents were told that there appeared to be no connection between my eyes and my brain. They recommended institutionalizing me as a blind child. That was what was done in those days. Children with disabilities such as mine were usually separated from their parents and learned Braille and functional skills at Schools for the Blind. This early sequestering was true for many other types of disabilities, too.

My parents were Irish-Italian Catholics and reached out to family and friends for prayers. There was even a letter sent to the Pope by my aunt, who was a nun. What happened next remains a mystery. On Good Friday of 1954 at 3:00 pm, while I was still hospitalized, it was witnessed by doctors that I was able to see. It was medically unexplained. Of course, my parents believed that it was a miracle. I was subsequently discharged from the hospital and returned home to my family.

Mom and Dad never said a word to me about this, nor did any other family member until that birthday year on the bridge between

3

being a child and maturing to teenage years. It was fully recorded in my baby book, along with other milestones, such as when I smiled, sat up, got my first tooth, took my first steps, received vaccinations, and so on. My mother saved the cards with well wishes from friends who learned what had happened.

What was significant about being born blind was what happened a few years later. When I was six years old, my parents planned a long-awaited vacation to Niagara Falls in early August with the four of us children. I tried to be helpful the night before cleaning up our dinner meal. I offered to take the used large glass soda bottle to the basement for recycling. Somehow, I tripped on the stairs in my haste and fell face down onto the bottle, which shattered on impact.

The glass tore open my face in multiple places. A large shard pierced my left eye and severed my retinal artery. There was also a deep laceration on my right forearm. Years later, I realized that I had instinctively tried to break my fall. My right arm protected my right eye, and the glass that entered my arm left an enduring large scar. I could have become blind again.

I knew I had gotten hurt really badly as I felt the blood gushing, but I couldn't see anything as blood was flooding over my uninjured eye from other facial lacerations. There was intense, sharp pain, but it was not overwhelming, maybe because I went into shock. I learned later that the basement floor had so much blood on it that it would not come completely clean. My father eventually put tile over it all.

My mom must have heard the glass breaking and ran from the kitchen to see me trying to come up the stairs covered in blood. I heard her urgently call for my dad, "Vincent!" They bundled me up in the front seat of the car, lying on my mom's lap. My dad drove. He dropped my two sisters and brother quickly off at a neighbor's house and then proceeded to the hospital.

There was a volunteer ambulance squad in our suburban town of Valhalla, New York, but it wasn't stationed near where we lived, so my parents made the choice to just drive me to medical care. All I remember of that ride was asking my mother if I was going to die. I don't remember her answer. I'm sure she would have said not to worry. I think I passed out after that.

I remember just the beginning of arriving at the hospital's emergency room, with the doctors trying to determine how badly I was hurt. I remember fighting against them as they were trying to open my eyes. I think I passed out again, as the next thing I minimally remember was being prepped for emergency exploratory surgery. I had been transferred to the eye specialty hospital, the same one where I was evaluated as an infant. But this time, the news was not good.

I had lost a lot of blood by the next morning, and the decision was made to enucleate or take out my left eye in another surgery. I had what was called a ruptured or open globe, and my retinal artery had been fully severed by glass. They couldn't stop the bleeding. I don't remember all the other suturing that needed to be done on my face and arm. Maybe they did that when I was already under anesthesia the night before.

Treatment of eye injuries in those days involved the rest of both eyes, meaning that both eyes were patched under heavy bandages. I think they gave me some sort of sedative, too, as I don't remember too much of those days after my initial operations. Maybe that was a good thing. After a few days, I was sent home to recover, still double-patched, in bed in a darkened room.

My parents were given a referral for me to follow up with an ocularist after my eye socket had enough healing time to custom-fit a prosthetic eye. I wore a patch after the initial bandages came off. I do remember lying in my bed in my room, thinking that when I woke up each morning over and over, I might be able to see through my injured eye. This, of course, was impossible. It was something that I just needed to accept and so were my parents. And I did accept it.

Darkness in itself was not scary to me. Black actually became my favorite color for a while. I even had a black dress. I was told a minimum of information, and that was it. I just waited to see what would happen next.

There were a series of appointments with the ocularist at the hospital in New York City. He showed me and my parents a tray of artificial eyes. It was kind of amazing that there were so many colors within the irises in those eyes. I told the ocularist that I wanted a pink eye. It was disappointed to hear that the eye that he would craft for me would be similar in color with my uninjured eye- brown.

It hurt when he poured what felt like concrete into my eye to make the mold. I learned the official term was methyl methacrylate, a plastic acrylic. The point was made that in 1960, artificial eyes were no longer made of glass. The process involved not just getting the size and shape right but also eventually coloring the iris, pupil, and surrounding white area (conjunctiva in an intact eye) to resemble my other eye.

This is where the artistry came in. The ocularist was able to make tiny blood vessels on the surface of the eye. I was surprised to learn that I would need additional prosthetic eye replacements as I grew, and of course, regular eye polishings to keep the surface smooth. Those future appointments were ones that I would not disclose beyond my parents. How do you explain to others why your eye needs to be polished?

Even when the eye was finished, there was an adjustment period. My socket would become inflamed and have a discharge almost constantly. Wearing an artificial eye is irritating, like sandpaper, whenever you blink, and it is worse with any dried secretions.

My dad was the one who learned how to take my eye out, clean it, and then reinsert it. He used a little rubber suction cup device. I learned how to do the removals and insertions by myself very quickly as I could tell that it was hard for him to do this. He didn't want to hurt me. He never complained or talked about it, but I can only imagine having to do this for a child. The ocularist made this easier for me by placing a tiny red dot at the top of the prosthesis to make it easier to know which way it had to go.

There were several more surgeries, seven in total, that were scheduled for reconstruction to correct my left eye ptosis (droopy eyelid). Apparently, the glass had severed muscles and nerves around my eye in addition to the actual globe. The anesthesia was horrible. They put a black rubber mask over my nose and mouth and administered ether. It smelled just awful.

Pediatric wards in hospitals were dismal places in the 1960's. You were committed to a crib for surgeries until you were about 10 years old. Lights went out early in the evening, and you were left alone in a ward with lots of other kids. Parents were not permitted to stay with children, and toys were not allowed. For one of my surgeries, my mom had left me with some paper dolls. A janitor yelled at me when one of them slipped through the rails of my crib and fell to the floor.

I heard the doctors and nurses talking as they made morning rounds. My eye loss was due to a traumatic injury. There were a number of children also hospitalized with me that instead had lost one or both eyes to retinoblastoma, a type of eye cancer that tends to spread from one eye to the other. They wound up blind. I knew instinctively not to complain as their conditions were so much worse. What was interesting is that they accepted their fate as well and didn't cry or complain, other than during changes of bandages. The worst part was when the doctors pulled off the adhesive tape that extended into our hairlines.

It took time, but I learned to deal with a loss of depth perception and to be careful not to bump into everything on my left side that I couldn't see. The upside of such an injury was the discovery that I could read at least twice as fast as everyone else. My brain didn't have to go through the processing of seeing and interpreting two images from two eyes. This gift was one that helped me with reading assignments, testing, and writing in school. Because my left eye could not close completely due to the injury and surgeries, I learned that I could sleep in class, and my teachers all thought that I was awake.

Thirteen is an impressionable age, so to be told about being born blind and knowing all that happened after that made me think about what I would do with the sight that I had and my life going forward. It definitely prepared me for wanting to be part of the world of healthcare. I did feel destined to make my life meaningful and not to take anything for granted.

Being a patient makes you a more empathic caregiver as you understand what it is like to be afraid, alone, and feeling like you are in a foreign land. You don't speak the language or understand the culture. My early experiences shaped the rest of my life. I felt that it was all part of a master plan.

Growing Up in a Large Family

I knew that my childhood was a very different experience than that of my classmates and friends. As the second oldest in a large family with nine children, there were responsibilities for everything from household maintenance- cooking, laundry, cleaning, gardening, animal care, and of course helping to care for the younger children. There was a range of seventeen years from the oldest to the youngest.

I learned how to change diapers (cloth in those days held in place with those big diaper pins and rubber pants), to warm up and feed babies their bottles (sterilized in a special bottle pot), spoon-feed the younger ones, supervise baths, help them with school homework, play games and read books together.

Because my older sister, Rita, suffered from rheumatic heart disease when she was thirteen years old, she was restricted from any strenuous activities. As the next oldest, even though I was a girl, I assumed additional responsibilities and learned how to help my father paint, tile floors, ride a tractor, plant bushes and grass, and a host of other skills which served me well in life.

Corporal punishment was real in our family. We received spankings, were put in corners, and suffered from verbal abuse, too. There was no child abuse hotline in those days. I learned quickly how to mostly stay out of trouble by just doing what I was told, even though I felt like being a rebel.

To accommodate us all, our family car was initially a black and white Pontiac, then a Volkswagen bus, and eventually a station wagon. It wasn't until the late 60s that lap and shoulder seatbelts were included in vehicles. As an infant, my mother's car had skidded on an icy road over a bridge, and I rolled out the side door down a hill. Having been cushioned in a snowsuit and a blanket on the front seat, I was found unhurt.

Even in the VW bus, if you didn't secure the door well, it would slide open on a curve imperiling whoever was seated near it. There was no such a thing as child safety seats. Instead, infants were positioned on the laps of occupants. Toddlers could be placed in a metal seat contraption that was hung over a seat but that did not offer any real safety.

My family had an assortment of healthcare issues, and I paid attention to how they were managed. This included five of my younger siblings suffering from varied degrees of asthma, requiring nebulizer treatments, humidifiers, oral medications, and allergy shots. Because of this, I learned to assess breathing and could detect early signs of struggle and wheezing. Administering injections for allergies was scheduled for select Saturday mornings, and my mother, who was trained as a nurse, taught me how to give them too.

When I was a teenager, my parents would drive to Florida to visit my grandparents and leave me in charge of the family. One year, six of my younger brothers and sisters got chickenpox simultaneously. My parents returned to see my **Quarantine** sign on the door. I had managed to treat fevers and place calamine lotion on the spots of my siblings.

Our family expanded year by year with more siblings. Eventually, there were nine of us kids. I learned a lot about healthcare by observing and caring for my brothers and sisters while growing up. Illnesses tracked through our household, affecting us, one after the other. I myself had chickenpox, mumps, measles, and, of course, flu.

We had a family doctor, and in the event that one or more of us got really ill on off-hours, he came to our home with his mysterious black bag, stethoscope, and calming demeanor. I only needed his services once when I became really ill with the flu.

Most of my siblings were not medically inclined. In fact, my brother, Aldo, would faint at the sight of his own blood, even if it was a minor finger injury. My other brother, Blaise, was interested in how his own body functioned, but in a weird way. This included one experiment in which he refused to "waste time" on something as menial as regular bowel movements. Of course, he became constipated after several days of his trial. It was no surprise when he decided to become a doctor.

When I was in high school, the nuns gave us four choices for young women. We could become secretaries, teachers, nurses, or get married and be homemakers. There was a hard glass ceiling present. Classes were offered for typing and home economics, neither of which my parents would allow us to take. Instead, we learned typing during summer break and grew up learning to cook and sew. I found it amusing that the girls who took home economics my senior year in my Catholic High School made bathing suits. They apparently did not use strong enough material or thread, as the suits fell apart on their first trip to the beach.

No one talked about sex- our parents or our teachers, the nuns. We knew there was a difference in anatomy between my brothers and sisters, but not why. Books were screened for 'appropriateness' in libraries and schools, and there were no sex education classes or television shows to explain anything.

Instead, there was a focus on what to wear and avoid and what was 'ladylike'. I was totally perplexed about why I should start wearing a bra, for example, or what 'becoming a woman' meant. There were whispers in my all-girls high school by my classmates, with questions asked and unanswered. I remember one of them being, "Can a girl get pregnant if you are in a pool with a boy? Even in college, we were shown a horrific film about giving birth but nothing about pregnancy itself. Needless to say, it was a bit of a shocker to finally learn what it was all about.

Hitchhiking was a common thing in the 1960's, as most young people did not own a car. It was frowned upon for young women, though, but again it was not explained. Instead, there were mysterious stories about being abducted and murdered.

There was tremendous emphasis on remaining a virgin until marriage if you were Catholic. We were told to always keep our clothes on when finally dating. Girls who didn't were shamed terribly. I knew that I didn't want so many children myself, as I strongly felt that you needed your parents as much when you were a teenager as when you were small.

Thankfully, the pill became available, and I secretly walked miles to Planned Parenthood to seek it out before getting married. That was one of the more embarrassing incidents ever, as the doctor who examined me called the staff into my room and exclaimed, "Look, here is a virgin! I thought I would die, but I needed to go through the process to get a prescription.

I found it crazy that my mother again thought she was pregnant when my sister and I were planning our double wedding. She would have been nine months pregnant by the date already set. She was relieved to find out that instead; she was entering menopause, although she didn't tell us that until years later.

An Interest in Healthcare

My dad was a civil engineer, and my mom was a nurse. I used to sneak peek into her books and marvel at all the various procedures and terms. I wondered where all the tubes inserted into a person's body went and what they were for. My mom did love being a nurse; however, she was not supportive of me following in her footsteps.

She complained about the hours, having worked evening and nightshifts for much of her career. The pay was also inadequate. Her own father was not proud of her desire to pursue nursing, stating that nurses were not respected. It was considered a lowly profession to be part of- almost like being a prostitute when caring for the basic needs of men and women.

But she understood that I wouldn't be swayed from learning more about such a career. I loved the white uniforms, nursing caps and pins, and the whole concept of helping people to feel better. Nursing was made more glamorous with television shows like Dr. Kildare starring Richard Chamberlain, my favorite.

I had always been interested in hospitals, perhaps because of the number of surgeries that I personally had endured from my early childhood accident. I would play "hospital" in the basement of our home as a favorite pastime, lining up dolls and stuffed animals in makeshift beds and bandaging them or giving them medicine.

There was a limit as to what I could actually do for them based on what I knew about care from my own hospital experiences. Now, they would call this play therapy. It didn't matter. My dolls always got "better" from my loving care and from dispensing those sugar candy dots peeled off paper as pills.

Our family grew as I did. By 1960, there were four of us children, including my two other sisters and one brother. We were lucky that we were able to travel internationally when I was seven years old. My dad was awarded a fellowship to teach civil engineering at Al-Hikma University in Baghdad, Iraq, for a year. We all got thirteen different immunizations to prepare us. The three of us girls attended U.S. embassy schools, and my brother went to a French preschool. My dad's students took us on adventures into the city markets and the surrounding desert. It was very different living in Baghdad compared to the United States. The standard of cleanliness was not as strict as what we grew up with. My mom boiled our water and thoroughly cooked our food.

I remember seeing men who were blind from Trichinosis, a parasitic disease caused by roundworms that could invade the body from undercooked meat. Life wasn't easy for them. They weren't institutionalized but instead became beggars. I realized that some people had a much harder life. Hospitals relied on families to provide basic care and nutrition for those who required acute medical care. There were open wards, and staffing was limited. I only got a limited view of this because of my age, but I heard my parents talking about what they witnessed.

I started volunteering at Burke Rehabilitation Center in Mamaroneck, New York, on weekends, school holidays, and summer breaks. You had to be a minimum of 14 years old to be considered. We were called candy-stripers because of the pink and white striped jumpers we wore over a white blouse accompanied by white sneakers. After 100 hours of service, we were awarded a cap and a small pin of Florence Nightingale's lamp, which we could attach to our badge. This was a prized achievement.

My younger sister, Teresa, accompanied me for part of one of the summers; however, she quickly discovered that it was not interesting to her. The only thing that she liked to do was to enter the temperatures of patients into their charts. She pursued a business career instead. I enjoyed and craved the whole experience. I realized that to identify what career you might be interested in, it was helpful if you could "try it out".

There were always new things to learn in that environment. They did not allow us to do very much usually filling water pitchers, running errands, helping to feed people, transporting patients to their therapy sessions, and delivering mail and flowers. It didn't matter. I was happy to be assigned any task. I was assigned to various wards and eventually to the Physical Therapy Department to volunteer. I loved it all.

There were other students who volunteered, but it seemed that they just wanted to socialize with each other. One of them tried to convince me to try smoking, but I declined.

Burke Rehabilitation Center was a great place to work and a hopeful one, as everyone worked hard, and we saw improvements in our patients. It was my first exposure to brain and spinal cord injuries, amputations, orthopedic conditions, and the effects of having diseases like Parkinson's, strokes, multiple sclerosis, and others. Recovery was always an incremental process and exhausting for the patients.

They would have multiple therapy sessions in a day, including physical therapy, occupational therapy, and speech therapy. Some of the patients had suffered traumatic brain injuries from horrific car crashes or spinal cord injuries from diving accidents. It was tough for them as they were often totally dependent when they were first transferred to the rehab center.

I was able to assist in both the Physical Department and the associated large gym volunteering during the summers of my high school years. Eventually, they hired me as a Physical Therapy Assistant. I happily rotated through the various specialty teams of Orthotics and Prosthetics, Traumatic Brain Injuries, Spinal Cord Injuries, Strokes, and rehabilitation for patients with other disease conditions.

I witnessed teenagers, some even my own age, who had been in horrible car crashes and became paralyzed and then faced a long journey through rehabilitation. The apparatus fascinated me-crutches, canes, wheelchairs, tilt tables, parallel bars, and paraffin baths. I learned how difficult it was for many of those patients to become mobile again

I got serious about a career decision when I was fifteen. My dad got hit in the head by a falling branch as he was cutting down a large tree. The nearest hospital was quite a drive away in the Catskills, and calling an ambulance just wasn't an option as the all-volunteer squad was nowhere near the farm.

My mom, a nurse but the only available driver, directed me to sit in the back seat, putting firm pressure on my dad's head wound as he lay across my lap. I knew this was serious from all the blood and the way I could feel his skull through the towel under my fingers. We made it to the hospital, and a staff member got him inside immediately. My legs were shaking, and I felt dizzy, yet relieved that he had survived the journey. I remember thinking that it would be a good thing to learn how to manage such a situation without being so scared.

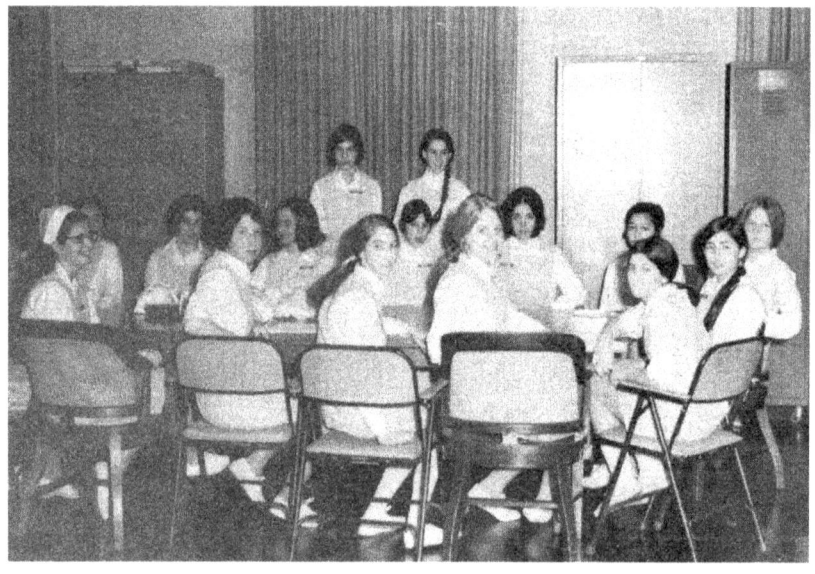

Candy-striping Days (I'm in the first row on the left)

College Experience

It was inspirational to help people become as mobile as possible again. So, I decided on a Physical Therapy career at Russell Sage College in Troy, New York. The school was top-rated for its curriculum and clinical affiliations. I chose a heavy schedule with the prerequisites that everyone had to complete, and then added science courses like Microbiology, Organic, Inorganic and Biochemistry, Physics, Nutrition, and others. These all had labs in addition to the classroom lectures. In addition, I also took Sociology and Psychology courses- beyond the basic course including Child Psychology and Abnormal Psychology.

Being two years younger than my freshman dormmates (it was a Catholic school thing to advance grade levels) was an experience unto itself. The sounds of Colour My World by the band Chicago resonated on my floor from stereos that others had. It seemed like almost everyone was consumed by wanting to go to parties and drinking. The very first night after arriving, the dorm emptied out towards downtown Troy to the various bars.

Being only 16 years old, I was not old enough to join them, even though I could have been given alcohol without anyone checking my age. I remember being awakened late that night and on subsequent weekends to the sound of loud retching along the outdoor pathway leading back to our dorm and on subsequent weekends.

There were continual invitations to fraternity parties at nearby Rensselaer Polytechnic Institute (RPI) and 'panty raids' of female dorms that occurred. Streaking was a thing in 1970 and even in nippy weather, there were always willing volunteers, usually intoxicated ones.

It seemed like there were endless conversations about the attributes of male students from nearby universities. One of the girls I knew took advantage of men who would take her out to dinner. By October, a number of freshman girls had already matched up with partners, even proclaiming them as their future husbands. There was also a lot of crying when their intended abandoned them for someone else.

I took advantage of the weekend activity patterns of others to appreciate being able to do my wash uninterrupted in the dorm's laundry room with access to all of the machines. It was a quiet 'white noise' kind of place to read and study in addition to the upper floors of the library. I also found a piano in a little-used hall that I could play to my heart's content.

I did join the dual university Russell Sage College-RPI Glee Club and enjoyed it immensely. I started dating an RPI electrical engineering student. He had a bass voice, which was novel to me, and loved music too. His dorm room even had an organ in it. We started dating, usually with a group of his roommates, all studying engineering.

VW bugs were popular with college students, and no one had a car that was expensive. In fact, in some of the cars, you had to position your feet on the sides of the floorboards to avoid the splash of rain or slush coming up through the holes from the roadway.

It became a regular thing to stop at Radio Shack so the engineering guys in our group could peruse and pick up parts for various class projects. The guys would be so engrossed by all those little wires and assorted component items mounted on peg boards throughout the store. It was a bit boring for me as I had no idea what could be assembled with such a mishmash of seemingly random pieces of equipment.

Thankfully, after this ritual, we would eat dinner at a deli-type place as part of our usual night out, which was fun as deli food was magical with big, overstuffed sandwiches, something I had not experienced growing up. I felt grown-up and sophisticated being included on those group dates.

That fall in 1970, all the guys received their draft numbers. This generated intense discussion of how low or high each of their numbers were what their individual chances were to be called up for service in the Vietnam War, even if enrolled in school. The television reporting was grim showing coffins draped with American flags being returned on cargo planes.

I had a "Big Sister" at Russell Sage, a senior named Ann, who was a nursing student. I loved to spend time with her and hear her stories about her clinical and what she had to study. I enjoyed the Physical Therapy curriculum but was still intrigued and a bit jealous of those who chose Nursing. Ann went on to become an Army Nurse.

We were encouraged to become pen pals with those in the service. Unfortunately, my pen pal soldier became paralyzed from an incident during a paratrooping exercise at Fort Bragg in North Carolina. I secretly wanted to join the Army, but my parents would have been adamantly against it. My education would have been covered, with the expectation that there was a service component to fulfill. I was okay with the service component and still wanted to seek out a military career. I did not realize that I could just sign up myself. Family approval was expected for such a major decision. It is hard to say if I would have been traumatized by becoming an army nurse and deployed to a combat zone. However, I do feel that I wish I could have had the experience. I was jealous of those who got to serve.

There was intense coursework at Albany Medical College in my senior year of Russell Sage College's Physical Therapy program. This included gross anatomy, which involved dissection of a cadaver. We learned the structure of the human body and how bones, ligaments, muscles and nerves all contributed to our ability to have movement, walk and function.

The rumors circulated before the fall semester began. There were whispers about the basement refrigerators that held "Typhoid Mary" and unclaimed bodies hanging from giant hooks that, in those days, could be used for dissection. A room that we were allowed entry into off to the side of our main cadaver room had shelves holding a multitude of jars with "anomalies" and "monsters." Many held babies with congenital defects, misshapen heads and bodies. It was the first time that I had ever seen conjoined twins. I was both shocked and intrigued that this could happen.

We worked in a large room with medical students who labored over their male or female-assigned cadavers. We had respect for those who had donated their bodies. The mostly male medical students interacted a bit with our mostly female physical therapy group. Six of us physical therapy students were assigned to each cadaver.

One day, we walked into our lab to find a six-foot-long penis of a whale deposited on a table near our cadavers. That was definitely a novelty that broke up the intense tedium of what we had to learn. Needless to say, my parents were horrified to hear this story from me. Truthfully, I think that they did not want me to know what a penis was!

It was not that unusual to discover anomalies in the organs and vessels of our adult cadavers, too. We found things like single or multiple kidneys, multiple spleens, and internal structures that were not where they were supposed to be. Although humans are similar in structure, it was fascinating to learn that there could be subtle differences that could be insignificant and unknown to the person until their autopsy. People can live with these anomalies, and sometimes, they are simply labeled serendipitous when discovered on scans or surgeries during their lifetimes.

Some people expire not knowing they had cancer or other conditions not listed on their cause of death. In those days, Cardiopulmonary Arrest was listed as a cause of death on certificates. We discovered the pulmonary emboli and coronary blockages that precipitated sudden deaths.

We dissected our cadavers over the course of a whole semester. In the end, their remains were cremated, and the ashes were placed into what looked like paint cans. I was impressed with all that I had learned about gross anatomy and immediately signed up to donate my body for science. I was later surprised to learn that many people did not support the donation of their bodies or organs for religious or just squeamish reasons.

Our physical therapy class was given the opportunity on Saturday mornings to witness autopsies conducted by the medical examiner at the hospital. This highlighted what we had learned in our gross anatomy class, but added a case analysis that made it all very real.

One specific case haunted me. It was a young man who was involved in a high-speed motor vehicle crash. He was unrestrained and ejected out of his car through the front windshield. When the medical examiner pulled back his scalp before he opened the cranium, we saw how his skull looked like a cracked eggshell. The reek of alcohol permeated his body, including when his organs were examined, and stomach contents sampled.

This particular autopsy happened after a night when my roommates and I had gone to a fraternity party at Union University. There was major drinking going on, although I did not participate in it. It was definitely not my scene, and I sought out the first opportunity to leave. The fraternity made a concoction of all sorts of different alcohol products, calling it a "hairy buffalo." I was not impressed. It seemed like very juvenile behavior to me, and instinctively, I knew it could lead to trouble.

A group of us decided to leave and accepted a ride back to our apartment. We crammed into this guy's car. I'm not even sure if there were seatbelts in his car. I don't think any of us put one on. We had to go back on the Albany thruway, and our driver (who I didn't even know his name) drove at least 90-100 mph. I prayed that we would get back safely, and we did.

That incident scared me enough to make a promise to myself that I would never get in such a situation again. However, it was reinforced by seeing the eggshell head of this young man who was similar in age to our fraternity driver. I never forgot that we did get back to our dorms safely. Such close calls forever stayed with me.

After my childhood accident, I had already learned that sometimes things are irreversible. In college, I felt more vulnerable in the world and avoided risk-taking activities as much as I could, especially after seeing the consequences suffered by others. I did not even know or understand all the risks, but I relied on my instincts to warn me when they existed.

Our second semester of our senior year focused on neuroanatomy and included lectures and dissection of a human brain. It was amazing to further learn how our bodies are assembled with small structures and neuro pathways that allow us to think, see, hear, smell, talk, feel and move.

We take so much for granted. It is not until a crisis when our abilities are threatened that there is a diagnostic process to identify what most likely happened in the brain for us to not be able to accomplish what we could before.

Undergraduate Clinical Affiliations

Besides the coursework and labs, my 4th -year Physical Therapy class rotated our clinical days with assignments at Albany Medical Center and surrounding healthcare partners.

One of the more memorable placements was at a hospital for children with complex disabilities. It provided institutionalized long-term care and was both uplifting and incredibly sad. The children did not have control over what happened to them in terms of medical care. Instead, they were dependent on an established system and a culture of accepted care. I appreciated the way staff at St. Peter's Children's Hospital got to know their patients with their individual personalities and abilities.

Affiliations for Physical Therapy were extensive and continued through the spring and summer. I was assigned to New York City at Montefiore Hospital in the Bronx, and then to Columbia Presbyterian Hospital on 168th Street and finally at Kings County Medical Center in the Flatbush district of Brooklyn. All of them were trauma centers with burn units.

I did not have a car and had to rely on public transportation using trains and the subway system to get to the locations. I laugh now at my naivete of carrying a small plastic water gun in my jacket to deter any possible attackers, but it did make me feel safe. Student dorm housing was included in addition to daily cafeteria breakfast and lunches. The cafeteria food was horrid. I ate breakfast as my only real meal of the day. They served things like tongue and tripe at lunch that I just did not want to try. Dinner was on our own, but I didn't have any money for food. I didn't want to ask my parents for such an allowance; so instead, I chewed on rubber bands to stave off hunger. I think I lost twenty pounds that summer.

Exploring the city on our own was discouraged as it just wasn't safe in 1974. There were even reports of staff being raped in the hospital stairwells, so I learned to join others when having to use them. July 4th sounded like a war zone as people were even exploding fireworks in metal trash cans. I was grateful that I had completed my time there before the Son-of-Sam murders happened in 1976.

Both hospitals offered a depth of hands-on experience and committed my career goal to working in acute care, specifically critical care. I was assigned to shadow a senior physical therapist on her rounds, which included the critical care units. She shared with me how uneasy she felt in such environments. All I could think was that these patients needed interventions soon after they were injured. One day, we walked past a room of a severely burned patient as one nurse was giving a report to another, including "another finger falling off." I hated that I had heard others say that the range of motion we provided would only serve to make sure that our patients could fit into their coffins.

Many of the patients had suffered multiple trauma in addition to their burns. I remember a young man who suffered an electrical burn while working on a high-voltage telephone line, followed by a fall of forty feet. Amputations were common, often from those who got pushed off subway platforms in front of approaching trains.

As students, we provided burn unit patients with a range of motion exercises and performed debridement of dead skin, often while the patients were submerged in these huge metal baths. It was several years later, when I worked at other burn centers as a nurse, that I realized how the windows were often *open* in the wards and debridement areas in New York City. Infection is one of the biggest challenges for burn patients. However, the open windows apparently were not a big contributor to this complication as the units had great reputations.

The clincher, for me as a student, was performing chest physical therapy on patients but was not able to suction them as that skill was to be performed by nursing. I felt limited by what I could accomplish. I also began to realize that the healing process was not just physical but involved recovery emotionally, too. It no longer seemed enough to help someone become mobile again or to regain function. I wanted to be able to help people to heal their whole bodies more fully. I decided to pursue nursing as a supplemental career.

PART TWO
Nursing Stories 1974-2020

Transitions 1974-1976

My family was shocked as they thought it was a step backwards in pay and prestige compared to being a Physical Therapist. I found a school, the Lienhard Graduate School of Nursing at Pace University in Pleasantville, New York. They accepted my undergraduate science course credits and applied them to be accepted into their two-year program towards a master's degree in nursing (MSN) and classes toward certification as a nurse practitioner.

After my college graduation, I moved back home to begin the graduate nursing program. This meant readjusting back to a busy family life with all the associated responsibilities of helping with housework, cooking, and childcare. Personal time was limited to late evening after helping my young siblings with baths, homework, clean up after dinner and bedtime story-reading. My study time began after all the chaos subsided and the house quieted down.

Working toward a graduate degree convinced everyone that this was a positive step for me. My mom warmed up to it quickly, having been a nurse herself, and took the most interest in what I was learning. I was genuinely surprised at how difficult the nursing program was. There was a lot to memorize, and it all meant something in terms of helping patients recover. If you didn't get the drug calculations right, you could kill someone. Learning to be a nurse was more intense than becoming a physical therapist.

The difficulty level progressed within weeks. We gave each other injections of saline, completely missing the interim practice of using oranges to mimic skin. This was followed by practice and demonstrations of conducting systematic physical assessments of each other. We listened to each other's heart, breath, and bowel sounds and performed breast exams. One of us volunteered to be the patient so we could all learn how to do pap smears.

Some of the early nursing 'fundamental' classes were fun. We learned how to make an unoccupied bed and then one that was 'occupied,' accomplished by taking turns as the 'patient' and the 'nurse.' We had one male nursing student in my class of 47 who confessed that he had never even made his own bed at home! Then, we worked on taking vital signs and becoming skilled with using a stethoscope.

My best friend, Gail, was often my partner, and I reciprocated. The ultimate test was when I practiced passing a nasogastric tube on her. She was a brave person who trusted me to do this!

There were classroom hours and clinical days. We were assigned through rotations in the departments of various hospitals in Westchester County and then in New York City. Having come from a large family, my pediatrics rotation was easier for me than it was for my classmates. That was only until I cared for a 14-year-old dying from leukemia and felt emotionally helpless.

I never saw a "normal" delivery during our OB rotation. Instead, there were twelve-year-olds delivering babies under anesthesia and women having their fourth child, all by different fathers by age 16. We had to do post-partum visits in run-down apartment complexes in which there were no working elevators, so the alternative was to climb rickety steps up multiple floors. I was bitten by "flying cockroaches" on one of those visits. The cleanliness of the hospitals in New York City was not any better.

An Ill-Fated Ripple Effect

I knew I was in a place marked by history, where people were placed away from everyone else- on purpose. One of my graduate nursing clinical rotations in 1975 was at a chronic care facility on Roosevelt Island in New York City. We were asked to carpool, as access to the location was very limited to one bridge. Almost immediately upon crossing, the island looked different from any others I had ever seen.

There were really old dark red brick buildings packed one after the other within a small area, only 2 miles in length and a maximum width of 800 feet. An assortment of names had been given to this location over centuries- Hog Island, Welfare Island, and finally Roosevelt Island in 1973. It was known for its prison and accompanying penitentiary hospital, a workhouse for petty violators, a smallpox hospital, and a "lunatic asylum". Our destination was the public hospital, Bird S. Coler, a foreboding place that honestly was also dirty and depressing. It was there that I met one of my assigned patients, a Thalidomide survivor who had been institutionalized since birth.

Thalidomide was developed in Germany in the mid-1950s and marketed heavily in Europe as a medication for insomnia and to alleviate morning sickness in pregnant women. Free samples were given to doctors to hand out to their patients with the written assurance that the drug was safe to take. By 1961, Thalidomide was being sold in 46 countries, and an appeal was made to the U.S. FDA to gain approval.

Thankfully, Frances Kelsey, a physician and new FDA employee, had read reports from Germany about the potential side effects of the medication and was concerned if it could cross the placenta in pregnant women. However, 20,000 doses of

Thalidomide had already been distributed in the U.S. as part of the initial "clinical trials," which were really just marketing for the drug. At least 207 of these U.S. patients were women, and 17 of them reported severe birth defects in their children. Dr. Kelsey refused the appeal for the drug to be sold in the U.S. It is now believed that there was an undercount of cases.

All of the affected women said that they immediately knew that something was wrong with their newborns in the delivery room when there was "dead silence" by all in attendance. Mothers felt guilt and shame that they had taken the medication.

My assigned patient was one of the U.S. cases, but also one of an estimated 10,000 worldwide. 40% of the babies died at birth, as miscarriages, or were allowed to die. Some parents could cope with a child born without ears, an arm or without legs and quietly raised them lovingly at home. Other parents deserted such children, as was the case with my patient. If it wasn't for the other cases globally, the public might have never known the scope of this tragedy.

My patient, Jeanine, was 25 years old and had already lived her whole life at Bird S. Coler Hospital. I found her in a ward of at least 30 other patients in a metal hospital bed surrounded by dull green curtains suspended by a metal frame hanging from the ceiling circling her space.

There was nothing that personalized her space. She had what I could only consider as a detached attitude- acknowledging the assistance provided but lacking in spirit. Perhaps it was resignation about her condition in needing assistance for absolutely everything, or because she saw an endless stream of rotating caregivers? Most of the patients there had no family visitors at all. They had been abandoned.

Jeanine was completely limbless except for a tiny, malformed, and useless hand coming directly out of her left shoulder. Demonstration of skills is part of a clinical rotation, and I was asked to perform a supervised dressing change on her wound- a large sacral pressure ulcer that went down to the bone. She was unable to even turn herself in bed, and a lack of good nursing care exacerbated her problems.

I explained to her what I would be doing, and she nodded her head. After gathering all of the items needed to clean and dress her wound, I proceeded to make a sterile field. My instructor was a very prim and proper older nurse. You had to perform well for her or face her scorn.

All was going well until a giant roach teetered off the curtain railing right into the middle of my sterile field. It was one of those moments that you were internally horrified but had to be very professional and just completely start over. The roach scurried off, and I went through the procedure. I was then assigned to other tasks for other patients.

My time at Bird S. Coler was very limited, and I did not get to return to Jeanine's bedside again as we were rotated through the facility. But her limbless and isolated condition in a drab medical setting with the cockroach intruding in her care resonated with me in an enduring way. Today, if she is still alive, Jeanine would be 60 years old. I can only hope that conditions have improved for those persons who are institutionalized requiring long-term care.

Social media has united Thalidomide survivors. A group was formed in 2016, and 15 of the members met in person in 2018. One attendee said that it was like finding "lost brothers and sisters." Survivors are still referred to as "Thalidomide babies." I realize now that my brief time with Jeanine gave me a glimpse of the consequences of the side effects of medications and shortcut clinical trial practices. The ripple effect of ill-fated decisions by those who just want to make a profit cannot be tolerated.

Montrose V.A. 1975

I was hesitant about a psychiatric nursing clinical rotation. The brain is such a complex organ, and I felt like I didn't understand enough about the manifestations of mental illness and how to manage them. My whole clinical group was frightened, too, so I wasn't alone worried about personal safety and my own insecurities.

The Montrose V.A. opened in 1950 as the largest psychiatric center in the U.S. The buildings resembled those built in both WWI and WWII and had a capacity of 2000 beds. Located on a sprawling campus of 210 acres, the buildings were all red brick and imposing to initially see. The movie "One Flew Over the Cuckoo's Nest" with Jack Nicholson had just come out in 1975, and the Montrose V.A. looked exactly like the movie. The ceilings were high, and the windows screened shut and bolted.

Our small group of nursing students was immediately ushered into a "locked ward" to receive our patient assignments. That process did not help me feel more secure because I was locked up just like the residents.

All were veterans, mostly from WWII and the Korean and Vietnam wars. Judging from what I had seen on television reports, I was sympathetic to what they had endured. Most of them were being treated for PTSD, depression, schizophrenia, and bipolar disorders.

All of the patients were dressed in tan hospital pajamas. Most were ambulatory and circulated between the hallways and the large community room. Even though there were lots of windows letting light in, there was a palpable general atmosphere of resignation, even defeat.

There was a locked nurse's station enclosed in glass where the staff, dedicated to their roles, seemed to congregate. Male orderlies had the most interaction with the patients tirelessly assisting them with bathing, dressing, eating, getting to therapy sessions, and shuttling them to activities.

Dispensing medication was a primary activity, and the patients lined up to receive the little paper cups of their prescribed meds. It seemed like many of the patients were heavily medicated, as their responses were dull. Was it a side effect of their medications that made them seemingly indifferent to our group of young female students?

Card games seemed to be one of the main activities for those who chose to engage in them. There was a TV that always seemed to be turned on creating its own circle of followers.

The vast majority of these veterans were smokers; however, this habit was a supervised one, at least in the section that I was in.

Some simply paced back and forth incessantly. The staff called them the "walkers". The most active of them could wear out a pair of shoes in a week. But did such intense activity calm their souls?

One person that stood out to me looked like he was a goldfish swimming. He held his body rigidly, leaning slightly forward as he walked. His arms stayed straight by his sides, with only his wrists moving in circles, as if he was propelling himself with fins in water. He didn't speak at all. Instead, he pursed his lips open and shut repetitively as if he was swallowing water or blowing bubbles. I wondered if he imagined himself in a tank given the restrictions of his ward, or did he feel transported to a large body of water and free?

We were told to circulate among the groups, and also to assess the general health of our assigned patients and identify any unmet needs.

I noticed that the patients varied in ages from being young in their 20's and 30's to those who were elderly. All were thin, and I wondered what their meals were like. Were they served institutionalized food or did the chefs take extra care to try to stimulate their senses?

My assigned patient, Paul, was young, in his early 30's, a Vietnam War vet being treated for schizophrenia. My interaction with him was fairly limited as he was scheduled for another round of electroconvulsive therapy (ECT). I accompanied him and a male orderly into a basement treatment room.

He was compliant, maybe heavily medicated to be that way. He offered no resistance and followed instructions. Had he felt better after prior therapy sessions that he just went along with lying down, being strapped to the table, and having the adhesive electrodes attached to his head?

The doctor inserted a bite block into his mouth and turned the electric current on. Paul's body jolted convulsively, and he lost control of his bladder. The 'treatment' seemed totally barbaric to me, and it was upsetting to witness. Paul was initially unresponsive but then seemed very sleepy afterwards. He was then transported on a gurney back to his room in the ward.

Since Montrose, I have cared for many patients over the years with mental health or behavioral health issues. Some of those that I saw with acute psychosis or street drug effects in the ER were more frightening than those I had seen at the psychiatric hospital. Those out in the community tended to be noncompliant with their meds and often attempted to hurt themselves or attack staff.

Training in crisis intervention techniques, including de-escalation methods were helpful. I quickly learned to not get trapped within a room with an unstable person, and to keep my voice calm.

I made sure that the ER that I eventually worked in had handheld metal detectors to locate weapons brought in by such patients. This occurred after an 80-year-old who had a psychotic break hid a large knife in his underwear and held staff hostage for a period of time.

Persons who had taken bath salts or Flakka in South Florida became insane and out of control. We received patients who ran around in traffic totally naked, lay on railroad tracks, or attacked others around them. One such person transported to another hospital bit off large chunks of his neighbor's face and ate the flesh while under such an influence. We had to give a crazy amount of medication to sedate such individuals. One man who had taken Bath Salts punched me in the face. I considered myself lucky as a coworker was rescued as she was being strangled.

I am so impressed with professionals who specialize in psychiatric care. I found it difficult to deal with people who were manipulative. Modern therapies are no longer as barbaric as they used to be, thankfully, but I continue to have a healthy respect to recognize those in need of support and will direct them to the resources that they desperately need.

Grasslands 1976

After completing my nursing program of study, I had to take an examination to qualify for a license to practice. I had a lingering worry about whether I had learned all that I needed to know to take care of persons of all ages with all sorts of conditions. The exam took place at the Convention Center in New York City. I really did not have any idea if I passed the exam. Thankfully, I passed the first time. I had completed all coursework except the clinicals for the nurse practitioner part of the program. The only available option was to shadow a midwife delivering babies on horseback in the hills of Kentucky. I instead wanted to work in critical care bedside in a hospital

My first nursing position was working the night shift, 11 pm to 7 am, in the Intensive Care Unit at Grasslands Hospital in Valhalla, New York. Its' history dates back to 1915 when it was used as a U.S. Army government hospital during WWI. In the 1920s and '30s, it specialized in treating adults and children with tuberculosis, polio, scarlet fever, and diphtheria. The age of the building was reflected in the cracking linoleum floors, high molded ceilings, and large windows. It has always been utilized as a clinical site for students who have gained experience in both acute care and public health.

I didn't want to work the night shift, being newly married, but that was the only option if I wanted to work in critical care. My husband, Don, and I had a small one-bedroom walk-up apartment on the hospital's campus. This meant I could walk to work, which was helpful as we only had one car. The only furniture in our apartment was a bed, a dresser borrowed from his parents, a kitchen table and chairs, and an old bookcase. This was supplemented by shower and wedding presents, so we had dishes, silverware, and everyday living items. Our budget was tight, and our only major purchase while we lived there was a new shower curtain.

There was a variety of cases we cared for in the ICU, including people both ill and injured. I learned to care for those involved in major motor vehicle crashes, fights, and fires and those battling heart disease, pneumonia, and a host of other conditions. There were also some more unusual cases, such as a pregnant nun who was admitted under a veil of secrecy for treatment of an undisclosed ailment.

Being a novice, I was assigned the more routine cases. This gave me an opportunity to watch the more experienced nurses' care for the "fresh hearts" coming right out of open-heart surgery and other complex care conditions. There was no formal critical care training program, so it was all on-the-job mentoring.

In addition to the hospital, there was a large jail on the campus. My ICU would receive patients from the jail, such as those who attempted to hang themselves. Even if unresponsive, patients were still handcuffed to the bed. I felt that I was growing up quickly seeing such cases coming in. My naivete about the world began to be stripped away.

The ICU was very sophisticated for the time period. We even had an intra-aortic balloon pump, which was placed into people whose hearts needed support pumping blood. Such patients needed to have a long knee immobilizer placed on the leg into which the elongated catheter had been placed through their femoral artery going up into their aorta. There were strict positioning guidelines to follow, the most notable being that the person could not sit up or the rigid catheter could pierce their aorta, and they would exsanguinate. I took such warnings very seriously.

For people who were too sick or unable to eat, a complex hyperalimentation intravenous drip was hooked up to give hydration and electrolytes. This was supplemented with intralipids, a milky emulsion, and also given intravenously in its own separate intravenous line. The emulsion would 'crack' if administered with other medications and could result in death. The formula was determined by the patient's labs; however, I overheard one of the residents prescribing an order for a formulation "to see what happens." Because it was a county hospital and many of the patients were indigent, it felt like some trial therapies were "allowed."

ICU nurses wore pink scrub dresses, which was the only time in my entire career that I wore pink. One of the male residents had a habit of pulling on the back ties of my scrubs to loosen them. Today that would be considered a form of harassment, but I was clueless at the time and just assumed such behavior was immature.

The night shift nursing crew that I worked with were an interesting and colorful bunch of women. They swore a lot, went out after shifts for breakfast tequila sunrises, and smoked pot at their parties. Don and I were invited to the get-togethers but left after not feeling comfortable with the general rowdiness, and we didn't want to put our new licenses in jeopardy if caught with an illegal substance.

My time at Grasslands ended when we decided to move to New Jersey, where we could buy a home in East Hanover that was affordable with a mortgage.

By 1977, soon after I left, the hospital closed and was rebuilt evolving into Westchester County Medical Center. It continues to remain a public hospital but also serves as a tristate regional trauma center and an academic clinical center.

My husband applied for a staff pharmacy position at the Veterans Administration Medical Center in East Orange. I wasn't even sure I wanted to work there, but I filled out an application as we still only had one car between us for commuting. Soon after, I got an official letter that started with "**Report to duty**."

I felt like I had been drafted. Since I did not have any other job offers pending since relocating, I decided to show up at the date and time listed on the letter. We had not yet made the move from New York, so we were forced to commute for two months. We both completed the additional paperwork, were officially sworn in, took an oath of service, and underwent a physical exam. Thus began my five years of service there.

By that point, Don's car, a Chevy Vega, had over 100,000 miles and was beginning to require daily oil replacement. One early morning, it was freezing and windy when we had to stop on the Tappan Zee Bridge. The oil was so cold that it wouldn't easily pour out of the container.

The VA and 7A   1976-1987

The Veterans Administration Medical Center in East Orange, New Jersey, was a huge hospital with1300 beds, the second largest in the U.S. The campus included the main hospital, a nursing home, a research lab, and some employee housing among, other buildings. There were layers and layers of bureaucracy with a process and forms for everything when you work for the federal government. I felt like there was not just red tape but every color imaginable.

In orientation, I learned that at my time of hiring, there were veterans from every war dating back to the Spanish-American war. Most of the patients, however, were from WWII, Korean and Vietnam era conflicts. There were very specific rules given- not waking veterans by touching them (if startled, they might involuntarily attack thinking you were the enemy), not wearing badge lanyards or anything around your neck by which you could be strangled, and a strict professional dress code. For nurses, this meant white uniform dresses, hose, and shoes.

My first duty assignment was to a 40-bed ward called 7A, a pulmonary floor with an eight-bed pulmonary ICU. Most of the patients had smoking-related illnesses, including lung cancer. Almost every patient required oxygen support, some needed ventilators.

I discovered that cigarettes had been issued to soldiers as part of their rations, and this led to addiction. To my delight, however, I met the Medical Director for the floor, Dr. Oscar Auerbach. He was already a legend to the staff for his research about the ill effects of smoking. He had a lab down the hill from the hospital with smoking rats. His work led to the Surgeon General's warning placed on the labels of cigarette packs about smoking being hazardous to health.

Unfortunately, they still sold cigarettes in the PX (the VA in-hospital store), and veterans who were ambulatory could go there to purchase them. Somehow, patients or their families were able to smuggle them onto the ward and sneak a smoke whenever they could. No surprise, we had fires.

I caught one patient flicking his lit cigarette into the bed of his sleeping roommate. Another patient went into his bathroom to smoke illicitly, but wearing oxygen, he caused an explosion. He wound up burned and did not survive. We had to evacuate the floor more than once because of the smoke associated with such incidents.

The staffing was the worst that I had ever encountered. When I worked the evening shifts, it was just myself as the RN and an aide for the 40 patients on the 7A side. That was it to pass all the medications, hang IVs and blood, change dressings, and suction those that needed it. Definitely overwhelming. But one night, the nurse called in on the 7B side, and all of a sudden, I was made responsible for the 40 patients on that side, too. I called the nursing supervisor but was just told to "do the best that I can." Apparently, you "can't sue the government," so they got away with such practices.

The V.A. was an academic medical center, and the best part was that it was a wonderful place to study. We were allowed to watch autopsies in the basement's large morgue on our patients who died.

There was one patient who expired for unknown reasons. I was able to carry his lungs with a huge pulmonary embolus back up to my unit to show my colleagues what had killed him. You could never do such a thing today.

The morgue was a chilly and creepy place. One of the pull-out drawers used to store the bodies was labeled "The Establishment." I was told that it was reserved for body parts. That did provoke some nightmares.

The patients were appreciative of all the care given to them, and their stories were endless. The staff became their family, as many of the patients did not have visitors.

I learned some new skills, like shaving men, and got pretty good at it. When you work in a pulmonary unit, you become very focused on sputum. I found that it became an involuntary response when someone coughed, even in a grocery store, to encourage them to "cough it up."

When the opportunity arose nine months later, I did request a transfer to the Medical ICU, which was more aligned with my career goals. It was another crazy place, but I was ready for the challenge after being groomed on 7A and having some very memorable experiences.

The VA is strong on offering training opportunities. I jumped at the chance to take their Critical Care Certification Course to learn more about hemodynamic monitoring and how to manage the variety of illnesses that were part of the veteran population. The VA had multiple critical care units, but the greatest staffing needs were in the Medical ICU. The patients were really sick, and all required advanced life support measures. That V.A. only had an "intake" area for arriving patients, not an Emergency Department. Patients who were assessed as critically ill arrived directly at the MICU.

Nurses had to work **8-hour rotating shifts during the day, evening, and night.** It was not unusual for them to work 16 hours or a double shift when help was needed.

Thus began my MICU experience.

Angel of Peace

Nestled securely within the branches of my Christmas tree each year is a very special handmade ornament. It is one of many saved over my lifetime with an irreplaceable memory attached to it.

Decorating the tree in my childhood home was stressful because of having to be so careful handling all of the breakable glass ornaments. I made the decision to avoid this pitfall after getting married and being able to decide for myself what went on our trees.

I never got into all the trendy decorations that others chose. My ornaments don't match each other. In fact, they all have unique identities and histories. My husband, Don, and I chose our first ornament together—a tiny crate of eggplants to remember the Italian restaurant we enjoyed going to on dates in New York City.

Our children made us an assortment of other decorations as part of school projects. Friends, work colleagues, and family members added to our collection when we told them we were moving from New Jersey to Florida and wanted them to make something handmade for us to remember them.

Some ornaments came from travel destinations while on numerous teaching assignments and national workgroups. There are White House Christmas ornaments from Washington D.C., a crayfish with a Santa hat from Alabama, a wreath made of wheat from North Dakota, and a miniature guitar from Nashville, to name just a few.

41

Other ornaments came from one-time-only visits. There is a little glass vial with pink sand from a Bermuda marathon location and a moose from Alaska. A decorated fishing boat from Nantucket commemorated our first visit to that beautiful island, which we then decided to return to seasonally.

Carefully unwrapped from its tissue paper each year is the ornament I cherish the most. It isn't much to look at artistically; it was clearly handmade. It was given to me by the loving wife of an elderly dying patient I took care of in the VA intensive care unit on a snowy Christmas Eve night in New Jersey.

Mrs. P. knew that her husband was not doing well over the course of the last few days. His heart was failing, as well as other organ systems, despite oxygen and an assortment of life-support medications. She appeared very frail herself, all wrapped up in a sweater and scarf, her white hair draping over her face when she bent to kiss him each time she arrived and left. She could no longer drive, so a friend dropped her off for visits and left me with a phone number to call when she was ready to be picked up again.

That night, Mr. P.'s blood pressure was dangerously low and dropping. His doctors explained to both him and Mrs. P. that they anticipated that he might need to be placed on a ventilator. He was aware enough to refuse such an intervention and stated, "I have lived a full life. Now, at 85 years old, I am prepared to die". His wife nodded her assent for "No heroics, Do Not Resuscitate." He became unresponsive a short while later.

Working on holidays is part of our job as nurses. People don't stop falling ill or getting injured to allow everyone to celebrate. The drama never ceases in an ICU. The noise level of monitoring equipment is persistent. Usual activities are punctuated by the need to emergently resuscitate someone in crisis.

But there was something incredibly peaceful about this one night. The hospital's hubbub had already subsided. The doctors and residents had finished their rounding and it was just the smaller night shift crew remaining.

The unit was full with every single bed occupied. We turned off the harsh overhead fluorescent lights, and only left on a minimum of small bedside lights and those at our centrally located nurse's station.

The ICU's large windows allowed us to see the softly falling snow illuminated by the outdoor ambient lighting of the mostly empty parking lots. Someone plugged in a radio and found a station with soft Christmas music. Time seemed to slow down.

Silent Night, Holy Night. All is calm. All is bright...

I moved a comfortable chair closer to Mr. P's bedside for Mrs. P. and put a warm blanket around her shoulders. Uncovering his hand, I moved it so she could hold it. I told her that even though he might not say anything to her, he most likely could hear her voice. I could tell by the fluctuations in his vital signs that he did listen to her. She told him her favorite stories of their lives together, usually preceded by "I remember when..."

I sat down with her to ask how she was coping. It was clear that her husband was fading quickly. When I asked if she had ever been with anyone at the end of their life, she said, "No." I told her that it likely would be a gradual process for him to pass away. His heart rate and breathing would slow down. She could stay as long as she wanted to. I reassured her that I would be there with her. She wanted to stay.

Sleep in heavenly peace...

Death did come peacefully for Mr. P., and I could tell that she was amazed that it could.

What was memorable for me was how composed she was. I asked her, "Are you alright? Is there anything I can do for you?" She answered, "No, he died so beautifully. I'll cry tomorrow".

Before she left our unit, she hugged me and then stopped suddenly to search her purse. "I totally forgot to give you this earlier. Thank you for being our nurse on this special night. I am at peace, and so is my husband."

That ornament, almost childlike in its' simplicity, is now 40 years old. It serves as a reminder to me that peace is possible even when all hope is lost. And Christmas Eve continues to be a sacred memory.

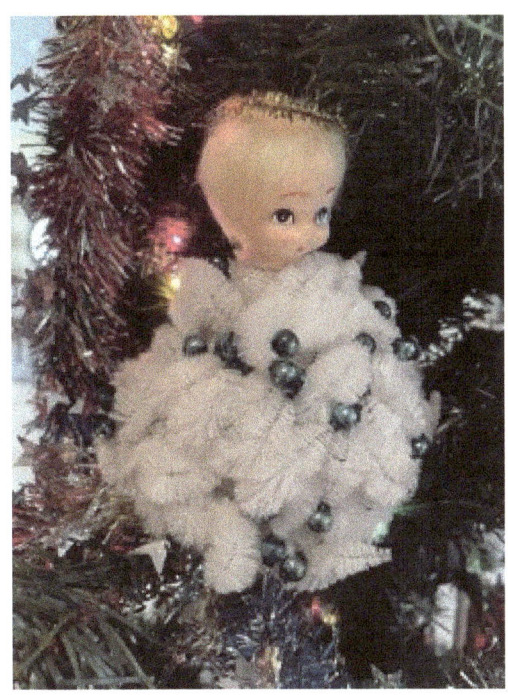

Trapped!

It was a typical busy night in the Medical Intensive Care Unit at the VA in East Orange. I was the charge nurse and supervised the care of the patients within the eleven-bed unit. Nine of those eleven patients were on ventilators. I had two patients of my own to care for as well. All were super sick.

At 2 am, there was a loud

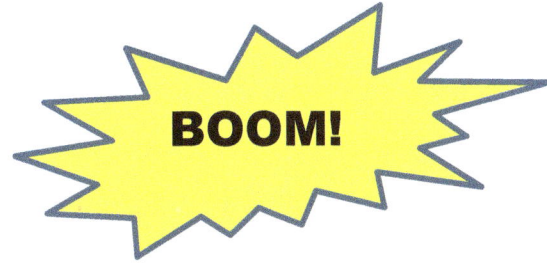

BOOM!

The building shook. We all looked at each other in shock and surprise. "What was that?" was my first thought. The noise seemed to have come from above us. I remembered hearing something about some kind of renovation work going on in the building. But wasn't there always some kind of construction project?

My unit was on the fourth floor of a nine-story building and, as typical of many specialty units, was located at the farthest point of a dead-end corridor. We began to smell smoke and heard the fire alarms blaring. Hospital fire safety training focused on the acronym RACE for **R**escue patients in immediate danger (where the fire is), pull the fire **A**larm (located right by the stairwells so you can access them on your way out), **C**ontain the fire (close doors), and **E**xtinguish the fire if possible (using a fire extinguisher). But where exactly was the fire?

Fires tend to be very limited to one specific area, so a major hospital evacuation is very rarely needed. The most common cause of fires on night shifts was from staff overcooking popcorn in the microwave or from patients who had been smoking in bed. I had already witnessed two fires at the VA when working on an oxygen-rich Pulmonary unit, and even then, we only had to move a limited number of patients, typically only horizontally, to an adjacent ward.

Unless the fire was on our unit, we had been instructed to "shelter in place" by closing the doors to our units and waiting until the alarms stopped. I called the house nursing supervisor to seek information as to what was going on. She answered, breathing heavily and coughing,

"There's been a generator explosion on the sixth floor above you. Stay where you are for now, but be prepared to evacuate your unit, just in case."

My fear level began to escalate, and my mind was now on overdrive. We had never prepared for such an occurrence in the ICU. How would we move unconscious, fragile patients who could not help themselves?

The corridor outside our ICU was now filling with thick smoke, blocking our access out to another part of that floor. A stairwell on one side of the dead-end corridor which offered a potential escape to a lower floor, but that meant we would have to get through the smoke and then perform a vertical evacuation with our patients and staff.

It was against every moral code to abandon our helpless patients. A niggling thought tugged at my brain. Are we going to die?

We were effectively trapped!

I quickly rounded up my coworkers for a debrief.

"Put wet towels down and seal the doors to the unit! Put the patient's medical record binders on each of their beds! Disconnect any equipment you can, like feeding tubes and secondary IV infusions! Have an Ambu bag at each bedside to bag those respirators! Get wet towels to cover your faces and those of your patients".

In a distant memory, I had asked a firefighter, *"How low do you have to get to the floor to decrease the amount of inhaled smoke?* "His answer was succinct. *"They call it a fireman's crawl for a reason."*

Oh boy. I looked at my five female coworkers. Two of them were Filipino, and one was of Indian heritage. All were petite in size and thin, which contrasted with our male veteran patients, most of whom were over 200 pounds. How were we going to be able to accomplish this?

"We have to get as close to the floor as possible to avoid inhaling smoke. Lower the beds to their lowest position. Lay blankets on the floor next to each bed. Get a partner and be ready to lift each of our patients to the floor! Someone get the flashlights!"

I could hear the sirens of the fire department beginning to arrive on the campus. The electrical power was now flickering. We had to be ready if our ventilators would cease to function.

I tried to reassure our staff.

"We are still okay here. Help has arrived. We can still breathe just fine. We should hear something soon."

The minutes ticked by as we continued to care for our patients. We tried but could not avoid worrying.

We didn't have to wait too long as the firemen cleared each floor and got to us. We were told that we could remain in our unit. Needless to say, close calls like that made me think. What else could we have done to be prepared? How on earth could we move our patients down the stairs? Do you go position each patient head-first or feet-first? How could we bring equipment with us? Where exactly should we go?"

It was a weird way to become a subject matter expert on emergency evacuation.

I resolved to make sure that we developed a policy and procedures to accomplish a critical care unit exodus, horizontally or vertically. One of my colleagues helped me put together a video demonstrating the rapid disconnection of equipment and patient carry techniques.

We expanded this work to include how to evacuate patients with orthopedic conditions, newborn babies, and psychiatric patients.

Together with a colleague, we published our recommendations in a critical care journal.

Within just a few months, emergency evacuation was included as part of annual training and exercises. Our maintenance department got me some dry ice to mimic smoke to make training even more realistic. I made everyone practice moving healthy people to safety over tile floors and carpet and down stairwells.

I continued this work when I relocated to Florida. We had emergency evacuations there more frequently due to hurricanes that would blow out windows and, in one Category 3 storm, tear the roof off our hospital.

I made staff work through specific scenarios like "How can you move someone who is in traction?" "What would the procedure be for moving a patient on an intra-aortic balloon pump?"

I still startle with loud noises, like a PTSD reaction. This story pushed me to learn more about emergency preparedness and response, and I wanted more training on how to train others effectively. There is nothing like a real experience to jumpstart a future direction of lifework.

A Journey of Confidence

Becoming an educator came slowly. As a child, I respected my teachers for what they could teach me. The smell of chalk and writing on an expansive blackboard in school was elemental and captivated me. However, I was intimidated to speak in front of my peers.

It wasn't until after college and starting a career that I gained the confidence needed to stand up in front of a group and talk. I wanted to become one of those exemplary teachers who didn't need to have notes in front of me but could just talk about a subject captivating those who listened. My dad gave me the best advice when I told him that I was nervous to be in front of a class. He said simply, "Just think about it as you know a little more about a particular subject than those in front of you". That advice served me better than imagining everyone in front of me naked, as was recommended by other educators.

I was driven to learn more about things that I directly experienced. That made teaching others authentic and real. What I hated were instructors that spoke in monotones and just read from their notes or slides. They lacked the 'hook' to make a topic come alive.

Working in critical care within an academic environment offered opportunities to learn and then share knowledge in a dramatic environment. However, I never anticipated the macabre subjects that would make me a subject matter expert.

Gastrointestinal hemorrhage, otherwise known as a G.I. bleed, was a frequent diagnosis in the Medical ICU of the V.A., and this spurred my pursuit of understanding what we were seeing. Veterans tended to drink heavily, admitting to a daily alcohol intake of cases of beer or multiple bottles of vodka. There were upper G.I. bleeds, and lower G.I. bleeds, depending on the location of an ulcer or tear within their G.I. tracts. Livers were compromised, which impacted clotting times and allowed bleeding to continue.

Some of the bleeds were unforgettably massive, with a river of blood running off the beds across the floor. These patients required multiple units of blood to be transfused, often through multiple IV lines. Patients could exsanguinate before our eyes despite all efforts. The use of Blakemore tubes with their integrated large balloons to provide pressure against esophageal varices was common.

The VA's medical library offered historical insight into why such conditions occurred and how they were managed over decades of research. For example, I read about the history of blood replacement as a treatment and was a bit nauseated to learn that volunteers had actually drank specific quantities of blood to determine how much blood might have been lost when emesis or stools changed color to black, maroon, or bright red.

I found that tidbits from such research held the attention of those I was trained. I supplemented information with making my own handmade life-size models of internal organs, including over 20 feet of intestines made from tube gauze.

This led to my recruitment to teach within the hospital and in classes at local nursing schools. Remaining clinically active afforded me the raw material to keep my material fresh and relevant.

Swimming Upstream

After relocating from New Jersey to South Florida and switching from critical care to the ER, I found my interest area shifting to a focus on injury prevention. I had already learned as a pediatric trauma survivor that some injuries are irreversible. Much of what we saw in the ER was predictable and preventable. It became my passion for doing all I could to change public opinion that such tragedies were not "accidents."

My South Florida hospital's location adjacent to I-95 made us a destination for some awful high-speed crashes. Initially, there were no designated trauma centers. Casualties came to the closest hospital.

People who didn't have their seat belts were subjected to life-threatening injuries during rollovers or if they were thrown from their vehicles. Many were ejected out of the front windshields, the rear window, the side windows, or even out the sunroofs, tossed like rag dolls strewn across the highway. The first question asked of an incoming rescue call for a motor vehicle crash was "Restrained?"

Sometimes alcohol was a factor, especially at night. Our local high schools all suffered student deaths each year.

There was additional urgency beyond increasing seatbelt use to the correct positioning and restraining of child safety seats. By the mid1990's, infants were getting decapitated by the airbags if they deployed while the child safety seat was in the front seat of vehicles.

The worst calls I ever had to make were to notify families of those injured. The three universities in our community had students who were both local and distanced from their homes. I could feel the dread and sharp intake of breath on the phone speaking to the moms and dads when I had to start with, "My name is Mary, one of the ER nurses at Boca Raton Community Hospital. Your son (daughter) came to us after a motor vehicle crash." If the parents could have crawled through the phone, they would have been there immediately.

I lobbied my ER director and fellow ER nurses to initiate a community injury prevention education program. This was a total volunteer effort in addition to working shifts, but it felt like the right thing to do to reduce the carnage that we were seeing. It was no surprise that I was asked to lead the program and accepted with some trepidation. Thankfully, we were able to be trained to use a new nationally developed program by the Emergency Nurses Association (ENA) for the schools.

The slides we used had all the statistics explaining how and why crash injuries occurred, but they also featured deidentified actual crash photos and showed the types of teenage injuries that could occur. A poignant addition included a video of a medical examiner doing a death notification. A letter was sent to our area high schools, and my small team of ER colleagues was immediately booked at all of them. There was no cost for our presentations as we were all volunteers. Our local towing companies brought crashed cars on each campus for the days of our presentations.

As nurses, we care for patients, focusing on their care one person at a time. It was time to join the movement to "swim upstream" and make a difference to stem the downstream tide of such devastation. The cost of injury was not just physical and emotional, but the 'bean counters' (those in finance) shared that it was cheaper to die than to live after severe injuries.

I applied to the Emergency Nurses Association to work with a small national workgroup to develop a "Crash Course" for Motor Vehicle Injury Prevention. This was another volunteer project, funded by the National Highway Traffic Safety Administration (NHTSA). It allowed for travel for meetings and being able to teach the Train-the-Trainer curriculum to emergency nurses across the U.S. Being part of a team helped to further decrease my anxieties to teach.

I was inspired to gain more skills needed to advance my teaching capabilities and applied to Florida International University for their doctoral program in education. Their motto was "to make a difference." That worked for me as my goal was to learn skills to further public education about injury prevention. There was also the reality that additional letters after your name gave credibility to what you spoke about. I began that program in 1993 and spent the next four years completing all requirements towards the degree in addition to working at the hospital. A doctoral program is called a terminal degree for a reason- it almost kills you. I would finish class by 9 pm and then work the night shift in the ER. I was the only nurse in my class.

In 1996, NHTSA awarded me my first grant to lead a Safe Communities project for my community as part of a national initiative to decrease the burden of so many people injured or killed in crashes. This was a data-driven project with a major educational impetus. I sought the assistance of Florida Atlantic University's College of Business and Research Center to download and analyze over 165,000 injury cases from my hospital, the Medical Examiner's office, and seatbelt observational surveys. My dissertation resulted in a systems model for community injury prevention that included new methods to profile and trend all mechanisms of injury patterns.

Business colleagues were intrigued that my "numbers meant something" as each of the cases in the database reflected real people who were injured. They got to meet some of the families, too.

I enlisted a team of educators that grew exponentially. We worked with lots of traditional first responders in fire-rescue and law enforcement as well as non-traditional community partners.

Margaret Mead, the anthropologist, made a profound statement in 1978 that resonated deeply with me.

"Never doubt that a small band of thoughtful, committed citizens can change the world; indeed, it's the only thing that ever has."

My most profound partners were moms who joined me at schools and told their stories. Together, we put "a face on injury" which is a very effective method to communicate the reality and personal impact of crashes.

One of the more poignant days was when one of the moms, Kathy, accompanied me to an entire school assembly at Spanish River High School, one with a history of fatalities. 2700 kids lined the bleachers of the gym. I could see them sitting from the floor all the way up, almost to the ceiling.

I started off our presentation with why we were there and what each student could do to keep each other safe. Kathy followed me, holding up and speaking about a handmade Valentine that her only child, Ryan, had made for her just days before perishing in a crash the year before. His last Valentine to her.

"I found this last night. I'm never going to get another Valentine, another Mother's Day card, or holiday with him."

She went on to describe how she still wandered into his room in the morning to wake him up for school or waited for him to come home in the afternoon, but he didn't arrive.

We both felt drained after leaving, not knowing if we made any impact. But it did. Within days after the assembly, a car full of students got in a significant crash, speeding while on their way home. But this time, the driver had turned around in his seat to make sure everyone was buckled. It made a difference. All of the injuries were minor. One of the moms who came to the crash scene said

"Thank God he listened."

My team and I taught hundreds of community presentations, both large and small, in all sorts of settings. These ranged from schools, Mom's Clubs, Rotary Clubs, Homeowner Associations, and Faith organizations. There were many memorable moments that occurred. These included teaching at a synagogue when the Rabbi's photo was taken down from the wall to make room for my slide presentation. One of our more famous child safety seat checks included Celine Dion's newborn. My mom helped me make a Ronald McDonald baby (a 'McBaby') for child safety seat checks sponsored by McDonald.

Grants also allowed us to purchase bicycle helmets in addition to child safety seats of various sizes. We gave these away for free at community events that included bicycle 'rodeos and child safety seat clinics. When the 6-year-old son of one of our ICU nurses was hit by a car and killed in front of his house while bicycling without a helmet, that mom helped me distribute and fit bicycle helmets for her entire neighborhood in her son's memory.

Standing up in front of a group takes confidence and bravery. But it can make a difference…

Props

There is an art to making a performance or presentation memorable. The theatre uses props to highlight a character or a background. Similarly, in the world of education and presentations, props can be the key to inspiring and motivating your audience.

I have always appreciated the phrase, "A picture is worth a thousand words". Maybe I am a visual learner at heart, but so are so many others who discover that learning can be embellished with something that highlights content. This was a goal I pursued in teaching. My focus had always been on injury prevention, so I searched for props to help communicate my talking points. Over time, I have accumulated a collection of methods and objects that have accompanied my lectures. I searched for greeting cards or real-life photos that I could scan into presentation slides that conveyed a message. Sometimes, these were humorous. Some were poignantly real. Cards have a way of saying things that we want to communicate in a creative way.

I tried to make statistics come alive. My clothespin display depicting the deaths and injuries from motor vehicle crashes wound up at Florida's state capitol to support a primary enforcement seatbelt bill.

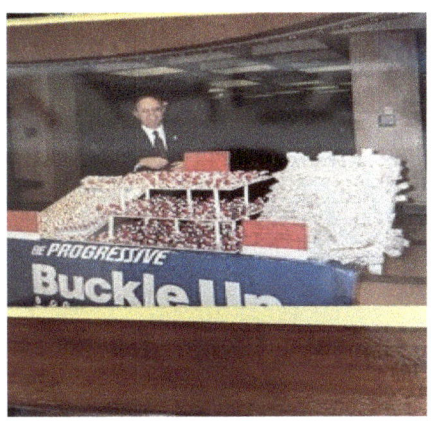

One of the first props that I liked to use was Humpty Dumpty. His story perfectly spoke to the irreversibility of some injuries and why there was a need to focus on prevention. I had a soft version for little kids and used real eggs for the older kids for an extra dramatic effect.

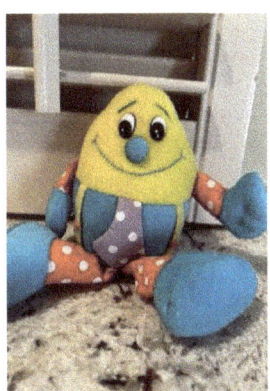 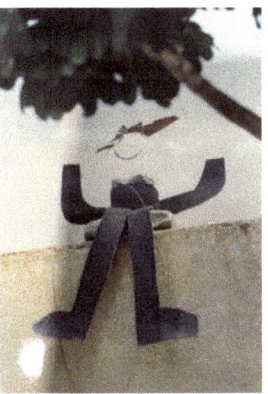 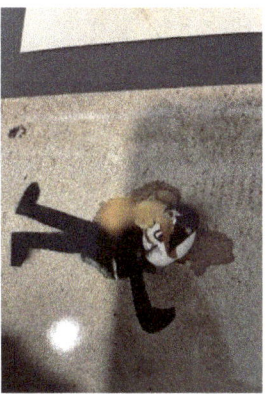

If I wanted to emphasize the protection that helmets afford for a multitude of sports, I brought a fractured helmet from one of our ER patients. He had survived a horrific bike vs. car crash without having sustained a head injury.

The helmet did the trick for him. I could also drop a melon with and without a helmet to demonstrate this.

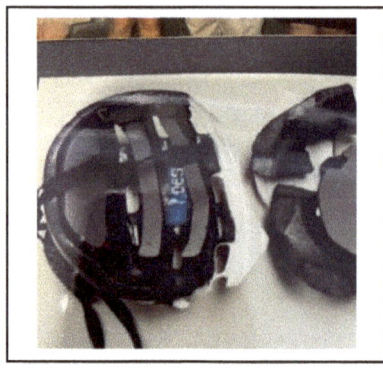

When I taught radiological preparedness, I would bring a Geiger counter and a piece of Fiesta Ware to demonstrate what a radiation source sounded like. Only the orange dishes have a radioactive coating, but they were a popular color of dishware at one point.

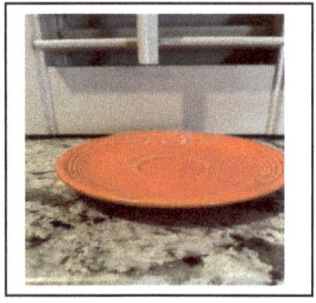

One of my adult healthcare students almost fainted when she realized that she had a kitchen cabinet with a whole set of these dishes. She felt better when I told her that she didn't eat her dishes, so she would be okay, but I think she still got rid of them after the class.

When there was a threat of protestors, I had to teach our ER team how to remove "Sleeping Dragons" from injured protestors trying to block traffic. A demonstration held their attention.

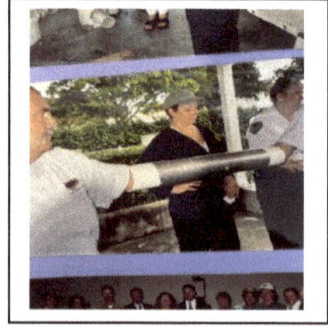

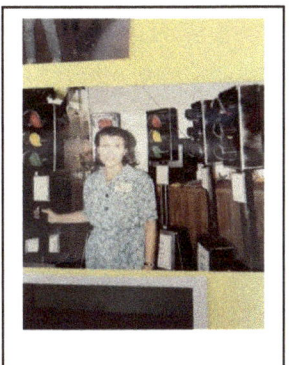

I have taught hundreds of classes on motor vehicle injury prevention and created a multitude of props including, for pedestrian safety. An example was making dummy foam board traffic lights to teach young children how to cross a street safely.

I would bring actual airbags that had deployed to speak on their protective abilities, but also the risk of placing a child safety seat in the front seat of a car, an occupant perching their feet on the dashboard, or a person sitting too close to the steering wheel.

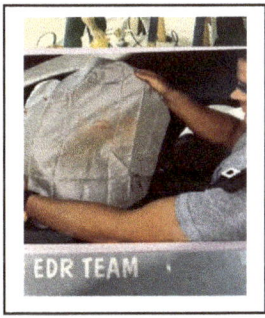

In the late 1990's, there were babies that were decapitated from being placed in front of such an explosive device.

Another prop that I used extensively was a set of crash dummy costumes, which I obtained from a small grant. These were popular on TV commercials, and I must have been asked a thousand times to loan them to kids as Halloween costumes (I didn't do this).

I would usually recruit high school students who needed community service hours to wear the costumes in conjunction with demonstrations and lectures at their schools.

One memorable experience involved two high school football team members who were desperate to fulfill their required service hours. They wore the costumes on a university campus with low seatbelt use. Their antics, dancing around and bumping into each other, attracted the attention of a reporter who somehow found out their names and placed their photo on the front page of the local newspaper.

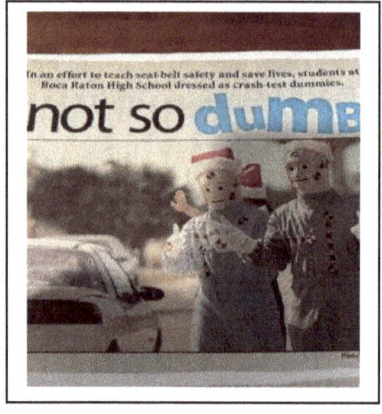

Per one of the mothers, they were totally humiliated about this, but there was a silver lining. Her son attached a clipping of his participation to his college application with the hope that it would enhance it. He was accepted into the university of his choice and, to my delight, went on to join the Secret Service, eventually guarding the Vice- Presidential level.

I had another crash dummy prop that was even more portable. It was a soft baby crash dummy with arms, legs, and a head attached by Velcro. It fits perfectly into an infant car seat. I used it to simply say to my classes:

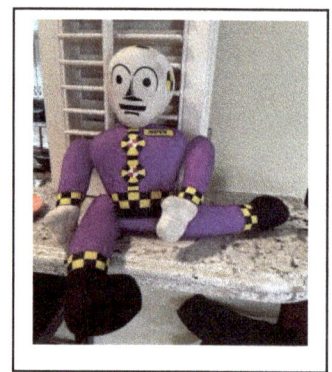

"In the ER, we can fix this (tearing off an arm), and we can fix this (tearing off a leg), but we can't fix this (pulling off the head)."

Again, this placed the potential irreversibility of a major head injury as a consequence of being unbelted in a vehicle. It always worked. I could hear the soft gasps from those in attendance. It worked as intended for Mom's groups, which I was invited to speak at as well.

There was one item that propped me up, though. I was nominated for a "Giraffe Award" given to "Women *who stick their neck out*" in recognition of my efforts to reduce the motor vehicle crash rate in our county. This was a simple paper certificate that was issued but became my most cherished award.

My friend surprised me soon after with a giraffe stuffed animal that had originally belonged to her young daughter, who had died in a car crash. She participated in many of our traffic safety endeavors following such a devastating loss. It was a sweet but humbling reminder of why we needed to continue working for community safety.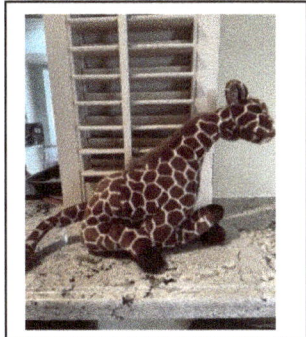

Props can come in many forms and benefit both students and educators. We all need such props as we teach our children, and then we can witness the affirmation that what we do can make a difference.

Burn ICU- Soul Searing

The worst burns go to burn centers. I have worked in a number of them over the years, always in the burn critical care units, always on night shifts. It is a challenging environment as the units become bubbles to protect patients from infection, a major threat.

As a specialty unit, burn units are referral centers for major burns of all ages caused by fires, chemicals, or electricity, on top of trauma associated with the injury- car crashes, high voltage lines, lightning, a fall onto train tracks, explosions. It was not unusual to receive burn patients arriving by ground transport or flown in from local or other states for the team's expertise.

Most people think of sunburn or blistered skin, first or second-degree burns, or partial thickness injury. Burn units see a level way beyond this: third-degree and beyond or full-thickness insults, sometimes to the point of losing ears, noses, fingers, or total extremities from tissue damage or loss of perfusion. Assessment for smoke inhalation is always done and may require being placed on a ventilator. Multiple surgeries are usually needed, and treatments can last for years in the healthcare system. Burns can have cosmetic and disfiguring consequences.

The first thing you notice when you walk into a burn unit is that it is warm. Thermostats are turned up as the patients do not have the available skin surface to shield them from air conditioning. When there is injured skin, cold can cause shivering and the loss of precious calories needed for healing. There is a room for staff to change out of street clothes into scrubs and then don head to toe personal protective equipment. Visitors are limited also to prevent infections.

Taking care of children was the hardest part of working in the burn unit. My kids were little at the time, and I felt for the toddlers who held up their arms, wanting to be picked up from their cribs and hugged. There was never enough time beyond a precious few minutes to just sit and play with them. There were medications to be given, dressings to change, suctioning of secretions, and on-and-on nursing care for the adults and children assigned on each shift.

But there was one baby that touched my soul and left a scar- an ember of enduring sadness that resulted in needing to make that my last burn unit case. One night, a ten-month-old boy, Tyler, was brought in as a 100% burn from a fire. The report from the rescue was that his parents were drug users. They had been drinking and smoking on the couch in their mobile home living room and had fallen asleep there.

Possibly, it was a dropped lit cigarette that somehow started the fire, smoldering maybe slowly and then consuming the room and very quickly the rest of their home. The parents woke up and fled the house, leaving their baby to burn until the fire department arrived.

The lieutenant who administered mouth-to-mouth on the child said that he felt his own lips burning when he was attempting resuscitation. Tyler's body was charred from the flames and the smoke, but he had survived. The odds against him were extreme.

Over the course of the next three nights, I cared for Tyler. Neither of his parents or any other family member had come to visit him, and this was heartbreaking. He was alone to endure unspeakable pain and surgeries in a place that was unfamiliar to him.

Having immediately been placed on a ventilator, I never heard his little voice. His chest, abdomen, and extremities had been surgically cut to relieve the building pressure of having endured circumferential burns. All I could do was to administer his pain medications and gently talk to him so he maybe subconsciously knew that someone was caring about him.

On the third night, Tyler was placed on high-frequency jet ventilation. At the time, this innovative device assisted with poor chest compliance. His body was progressively failing. Despite every possible intervention, he went into cardiac arrest. I'll never forget my fingers doing chest compressions on his tiny chest and sinking through the dead eschar on his sternum to the underlying bone. It was a futile effort to think that we could bring him back to life and that his life could be like that of any other child.

In some cases, it hurts too much and sear the soul within us.

During the Covid-19 pandemic, I recalled this story as my colleagues worked against impossible odds to be there for their patients, having to deal with PPE, especially when families were not allowed. Perhaps, we have our own internal burn injuries that accompany us through our careers and beyond.

When They Don't Cry

The proximity to water in South Florida is everywhere with the ocean, the multitude of canals, backyard and community pools, and even buckets, tire swings, and bathtubs. As a consequence, submersion injuries, including both drowning and near-drowning, are unfortunately too common.

Some of these drownings are intentional- people giving up on life and seeking finality. People walking toward solace in the ocean. Others purposefully drive into canals, causing not only their deaths but any unsuspecting occupants, often children, who are caught in the web of despair. And then there are those persons who are distracted or intoxicated and veer off the road into the murky water. If witnessed, they may be recovered alive. Some are found many years later when the vehicle is unexpectedly located when dredging the canal, by fishermen, or when the water level drops.

Baby drownings are the worst, though. Little ones just see the surface of the water as glittering and beckoning to them. Even if they have been with their parents before in water, it was always for fun, and there was safety in the arms of mom or dad. It doesn't take long to drown. Backs are turned, or those assumed to be watching the children look away, even if just for moments. Babies crawl through open doors, doggie doors, or simply fall into the shallow end, the deep end, or anywhere in between. One afternoon, we cared for twin boys. One scampered after a ball which landed in the pool, and the other followed right behind.

Sometimes, they are discovered quickly. Sometimes not. But there is always an effort made to resuscitate them. In the ER, we listen to the report called in by the paramedics. And hope against hope that they will make it to us awake. All is quiet as we listen for cries coming through the ambulance entrance. And it is music to our ears if we hear any signs of life. But when they don't cry, we struggle through our own tears to give these little ones every chance to survive. We breathe for them and warm them up with our machines as the parents' crumple near us, holding their little hands, so pale and cold and lifeless.

Sometimes, their deaths are called when it is known that they were down for too long. Because no one noticed they were missing. We cannot judge what happened. Some babies survive for a little while even though they don't wake up at all. Then they are declared as "vegetative" or "brain dead". Their loss is just as painful as their hearts continue to beat, but their brains are not functioning.

I have worked with nurses who don't like to work on kids with any type of issue. They get irritated when they are noisy or fearful. I tell them, it is good when we can hear them cry. Because otherwise we may just hear the cries of their parents.

Mr. Itchy   Memorial Day Weekend 1992

It was one of those horrific night shifts in my community hospital's ER in Florida. There were multiple cardiac arrests and traumas, with several fatalities. We had to designate a room off to the side of the department to place the bodies awaiting transport to our morgue. There just wasn't time to get them there for what seemed like hours. The wait times were also hours long for arriving patients with non-urgent conditions.

Not everyone was patient, and I kept hearing one particular plea in the background, *"But I'm itchy!"*. Being fairly new to Florida, I asked my colleagues why we had so many itchy people coming for help. The replies were puzzling.

"Every year around this time, it's a common problem. It's called sea lice. No one really knows what causes it."

Because this condition caused an itchy rash mostly under the bathing suit area, there was fear and a range of resultant diagnoses of venereal disease, chickenpox, and measles, or just diaper rash in babies. People tried remedies of their own including calamine lotion, witch hazel, garlic, athlete's foot spray and head lice medications. Out of desperation, some even used dangerous products such as fingernail polish, gasoline, undiluted bleach, and ammonia.

I like a challenge, especially after I called our county public health office and was told.

"No one knows what sea lice is caused by. We've investigated it many times. Give up trying to figure it out".

I'm not a "give up" kind of person, so I persisted with making phone calls and reading prior articles written about this phenomenon.

I was shocked to discover that there were reports of outbreaks and investigations documented since before 1900. Local fishermen from Cuba, Puerto Rico, the Caribbean islands, and Mexico were very acquainted with it, warning that they noticed it between the months of March through August. There was even an old folklore saying from the Bahamas warning about going ocean swimming between Mother's Day and Father's Day each year.

This was not a minor issue. It involved 250 miles of our southern Atlantic coastline and an estimate of over 10,000 people per year seeking medical care. Because Boca Raton juts out into the ocean, it turned out that our area was the geographic center for cases.

My ER even received calls from tourists with the rash who had visited our area and then traveled home from everywhere. Doctors from all over the world wanted to know how best to treat people. I couldn't give up.

My search led to a physician who was also interested in this affliction, and we teamed up on a project. We found professors in marine biology and a couple of willing students from Florida Atlantic University and the University of Miami who agreed to help us by growing cultures from our plankton tows. Wow, this was becoming fun and serious at the same time.

Our mission took us to the beach to interview lifeguards. They were so grateful that someone was trying to figure this mystery out. All of them except one had a history of getting sea lice multiple times a year, likely due to their routine of taking a daily ocean swim when going on duty. They agreed to blood titers being drawn and told us that they would put us on the Wheaties cereal box if we figured it out.

I submitted an IRB proposal to my hospital to conduct a survey of our 1500 employees to identify how many of them had experienced the rash and to complete a retrospective case review of ER records to determine how many potential cases there were each year, including recording clinical presentations. All of this was a volunteer thing done on my days off duty.

The team effort paid off. The cultures noted a preponderance of microscopic cnidarian larvae (marine animals with nematocysts or stinging cells including jellyfish, anemones, and Portuguese Man o' War). The biologists grew the cultures to maturity and were able to identify the causative organism- a thimble jellyfish! NOAA helped us to map the Gulf Stream currents to show how the larval jellyfish came closer to shore during outbreak months. It was all beginning to make sense.

When people swam in the ocean, the larval jellyfish got trapped in the mesh of bathing suits, and the stinging cells started firing with any type of mechanical pressure (sitting on the beach or on the car ride home, moving around in the suit) or a change in osmotic pressure (taking a shower at the beach while still wearing a suit or jumping into a pool).

People told us that they got re-stung when they donned their bathing suits again despite machine washing and heat drying them.

When I put out a request for such bathing suits, I received a whole bunch of suits, some still damp from recent use. My biology friends put them under a high-powered microscope. It was easy to see that the stinging cells remained active and could re-sting when worn again, even in just a pool. I found it interesting to remember hearing older people say, "Wear your oldest suit to the beach," as it became a recommendation to throw out a contaminated suit after getting "Seabather's eruption," as we now call it.

We published our results in multiple journals and did a series of press conferences. I received invitations to speak at Rotary Clubs, professional meetings, and schools. Besides my slides, I brought a thimble jellyfish with me, preserved in a small container to pass around. It was a fifth-grade student who dubbed my sample Mr. Itchy. Of course, our nudist groups insisted that if people did not wear bathing suits at all, they would not get the rash. This was true, and they had a field day with that fact.

This entire project solidified my desire to choose to pursue a career in research and to pursue my doctorate. Despite several significant additional projects over my lifetime, my tombstone will likely reflect the project that was the most fun and got crazy attention with an epitaph as the "sea lice nurse". I never got on the Wheaties box.

Shock Value

We heard him before we saw him. Everyone stood still as there was a loud, growling roar and blood-curdling screaming echoing from the direction of the ambulance entrance. It sounded like a beast. Visitors even came out of the patient rooms, their eyes wide open, to find out what would unfold. They didn't see much, though, as the patient was surrounded by paramedics and police officers and quickly ushered into an empty trauma room- mine.

The handoff was brief but enough to work with. The person who had called 9-1-1 was a female "friend" of this 38-year-old male named Joe. She was going down on him, giving him oral sex, while he was driving on a main road. His erratic driving caught the attention of police, who started following him. He was worried about driving with a suspended license and drugs in the car.

He regained control of his vehicle but then swallowed all the five one-gram cocaine packets in his possession in case he was stopped. The police never pulled him over, though, and he continued driving to the Best Western motel, where he had previously booked a room.

Shortly after arriving at his room, he started becoming restless, then hallucinating, hearing voices and was convinced that snakes were biting him. He started to get violent and began tearing up the room. This included wrestling the bathroom sink out of the wall and the toilet out of the floor. He then proceeded to throw the toilet out of the closed bedroom window, shattering the glass everywhere. After calling for help, the friend stayed until the paramedics and police arrived to tell them what had happened, and then she left the scene. She did not accompany him to the hospital.

Working in South Florida, there are many drug overdoses. Smugglers who ingest cocaine bags (cocaine body packers) can suffer the consequences when the packets spontaneously rupture. In this case it was more of an accidental release of a large quantity of what were poorly closed bags of the cocaine, causing a toxic release of the drug.

Joe was a big guy. Despite full restraints, he was thrashing his arms and legs violently and combatively while incoherently continuing to scream. He was grinding his teeth and spitting blood into his oxygen mask, having bitten his tongue.

Beads of sweat were running off his forehead and his clothes were saturated with sweat and urine. It took multiple doses of medications to begin to get him under control and complete a full head to toe assessment.

His arms were covered with tattoos, and I ended up placing an intravenous line between renderings of a grim reaper and one that read as KKK. There were more tattoos; the largest was spread over his entire chest- it said Hell's Angels.

When removing his pants, his left lower leg was grossly misshapen, with large areas of scarring over apparent missing tissue. As Joe became more lucid, he said that his injury was from a gunshot wound a year ago in New York City. The wound got infected and developed into osteomyelitis, resulting in multiple surgeries That explained what looked like a graft on his other leg. He said that he had chronic pain from this injury, requiring an implantable morphine pump in his abdomen, and needed a cane to walk.

But the biggest discovery came just a bit later when turning him to check his back. In four-inch letters across his back were:

FUCK YOU

I must have gasped when I saw this, which he realized and said, "Oh, you saw it!"

Joe was lucky to survive this incident as he was in critical care for an extended period of time in renal failure and requiring dialysis. He was a difficult patient for all who cared for him, demanding and downright mean. But he was also one of the more colorful patients to remember.

Extended Family

We spend 30% of our lives working, so it is no surprise that we have two 'family' groupings that we care about. Our home family is always who we want to be with and who we care about the most, but coworkers become our home away from home. Many become long-term close friends. Some refer to their colleagues as "my work husband" or "my work wife."

At a community hospital, there are fewer degrees of separation. We go through life's passages serially or collectively, completing our educations, engaging in relationships, having children, and caring for our parents. We also bond when sharing the daily drama or working in an ER. These experiences, while rewarding, also come with their emotional toll. It's important to acknowledge and support each other through these challenges.

In the moments shared before clocking in, during lunch breaks, or during a middle of the night lull, we talk about things both mundane and profound. You can try to leave your problems at the door when arriving to work, but that is easier said than done. All you have to do is to look at your coworker's face and know when something is troubling them.

We all knew that this one coworker was going through a divorce, but the day the final papers arrived, right before her scheduled night shift, it still shook her up. Hugs always seemed to be appropriate for tough times such as that one as well as for celebrations.

The motto in my ER was "Our family caring for yours". We knew the names of each other's kids and often had cared for them as they needed suturing of wounds, splinting of fractures, or assessments of fevers. We also cared for each other after miscarriages, motor vehicle crashes, and all sorts of illnesses and injuries.

We bond over certain ER cases. Often, it is because we have to face them together. One night, a coworker, Sue, went to check on why her patient still wasn't back from having x-rays. It was a fairly simple case- an intoxicated young woman who fell off a bar stool.

Sue came back to the desk white as a ghost and was unable to speak, just pointing at me to help her- to go to X-ray. I went there and was shocked to see our radiology tech raping the apparently unconscious young woman on the table. I got us through that situation, and we were forever linked in time, even though thirty years have now passed.

As many people as possible try to help with the most dreaded of cases, a "Code Pink," a pediatric cardiac arrest. We vividly recall every single one. Early one morning, there was such an encode from EMS.

A three-year-old boy had run out his front door into the driveway where a neighbor was picking up his older sister for school. No one realized the child had done this, and the neighbor backed up and ran him over in her minivan, crushing his skull. It sounded like a hopeless situation, but every effort was being made to save him.

I heard a gasp behind me from one of my fellow nurses, Anne, who ran into the room to help. She stopped short when she recognized the beautiful blond-haired boy lying motionless on the stretcher and his sobbing mother next to him.

"Oh my God! I know this family. They live on my street. My kids go to school with his sister."

Such a horrible scenario becomes even more real when family connections are realized. We directed Anne, who knew the family, to stay with and support the mom. The rest of us continued with the compressions, bagging, and pushing medications. The room was hushed other than orders being given and repeated. I will be honest: we all had tears in our eyes as this was a battle that we instinctively knew we would not be able to win. We could see a tire track traversing his head despite all the blood.

When the resuscitation was finally terminated, I left the room with a nurse staying behind with the mom and went to relieve and thank the agency nurse, April, who watched over my zone of patients while I helped with the code. That nurse was in tears, too. Why? She confided that she had lost her four-year- old in a fire several years back but was reliving his death with our latest case. No one knew about her history. But she became part of our family that day, even though she was with us only on a temporary basis. She shared our pain, and we shared hers.

There have been many times when I helped my coworkers, and they helped me. I remember having to lock myself in our breakroom bathroom to cry after I had returned from helping with an inpatient cardiac arrest on one of the floors. It involved a patient with glioblastoma, a malignant brain tumor- the same diagnosis as my sister, who was dying of the disease. My coworkers understood why I was upset- they knew about my sister already. It can be hard to separate work from real life when they are so intertwined.

It is apparent that we all need each other to get through work and to get through life. When there is a senseless tragedy, there are no words that can make it better. One of my colleagues was sobbing in our utility room, cleaning off the torn-off lower leg of one of our fatal crash victims. The leg still had the young man's sneaker attached to it. It had been found at the scene after he had been transported to us. Another hug, another bond, sharing the tragic loss of life.

Nurses, like war veterans, do not share the majority of what they have witnessed and been a part of. We just have each other's collective memories. We are not so different from elephants, I guess. We don't forget; we move on.

My daughter was very perceptive, even at a young age. She learned to just look at my shoes when I came home from work, to see how much blood splatter there was on them. She knew when it was a tough shift. My response was always the same, to hug her, my son and my husband, grateful that I had them to boost me back up.

I think about all the healthcare staff who have endured the seemingly unending pandemic. I can only hope that their "battle buddies" remain their extended family, their home away from home.

The Fear Factor

Both the public and healthcare staff get nervous when a hazard or potential threat emerges in their community or is highlighted on national news. It can be precipitated by an event of great magnitude, such as 9-11 or a local mass shooting. There is a fear of the unknown and perceived danger to oneself or to family members. All it takes is something even like a novel infectious disease.

I witnessed such widespread anxiety in Boca Raton during September and October of 2001. The nation was already on edge following the terrorist attacks associated with 9-11. Our concern grew locally when we learned that several of the terrorists lived nearby and went to our gyms and restaurants. But there was more to come.

On the morning of October 4, 2001, not even a month after 9/11, there was another drama evolving in Palm Beach County, Florida. At an emergency management meeting with representatives from police, fire, and hospitals, beepers started going off randomly around the room. One by one, each person got up and left the room to answer them. It was one of those 'aha' moments with a dawning realization that something big might be happening in which everyone was involved.

The beeper message to everyone was the same. There was a case of anthrax, an uncommon, potentially lethal biological illness, diagnosed at one of our local hospitals. JFK Medical Center.

The county health department had been notified initially on October 2 by an astute ER physician about the possible case based on a suspicious chest x-ray. The patient had presented with complaints of a fever, shortness of breath, and chest pain, but deteriorated quickly. An investigation was opened to determine the source of his exposure. The hospital's lab sent specimens to the CDC for confirmation that it was bacillus anthracis. Anthrax is considered by the CDC to be a Category A biological agent. It has a high mortality rate for the inhalational form, between 50-80%, even when treated. Bob Stevens, 63 years old, died on 10/4.

Bob was employed as a photo editor and worked at the American Media Institute- the home of several publications, most notably the National Enquirer, which is well-known for its sensational articles including about aliens and awkward celebrity sightings. A second AMI employee was diagnosed with pneumonia on the same day that Bob passed away. It became urgent to check out the building.

Evidence of a white powdery substance was found by the health department on 10/4 on Bob's desk and the surrounding floor. A suspicious envelope was identified in his trash and logged as additional data. A fire-rescue hazmat team responded to the AMI building in full Level A gear and proceeded to evacuate everyone outdoors. Employees were terrified and began calling their families. Everyone had to undergo mass decontamination, meaning stripping off all clothes and washing themselves head to toe to rinse off any potential deadly spores.

The media quickly got wind of what was happening. They had a field day filming what they could see of fire-rescue in their gear assisting naked people despite the meager privacy curtains placed around them. The entire campus became cordoned off by police. Multiple local, state, and federal agencies were spotted, including the CDC, FBI, and EPA.

Nasal swabs were taken of all the AMI employees. A positive result was noted from another person including her computer screen from work. Swabbing of various parts of the building turned up positive for spores in an additional 90 other locations. From our first responder community, we learned from the CDC hat it was a weaponized strain of anthrax- potentially for biological warfare. That was a "sphincter tightening" revelation.

Was a lethal toxin sent just through the mail or by other means? The word spread quickly, leading to panic among the community.

Were we under attack again? White powder sightings escalated to the point of being ridiculous. Talcum powder spilled on the floor, sugar spilled in a grocery aisle, and so on. There would eventually be over 3000 calls in South Florida to hazmat from fearful people. Businesses and homeowners alike were afraid to open mail and packages.

Bob's wife shared that he was near-sighted. He had a habit of taking off his glasses and holding the mail up close so he could read the contents more easily. He most likely inhaled more spores in that way when the powder leaked out, and that coupled with his age may have made him more vulnerable.

Because of the potential time delay in identification, prophylactic antibiotics were planned to be administered to potentially exposed workers. This included the AMI building and the mail processing facility that serviced it. A shipment of antibiotics was requested from the Strategic National Stockpile. This eventually arrived at Palm Beach International Airport on huge pallets. It took time for teams of health department employees to unpack the huge crates and get the product ready for distribution in packets of individual doses.

The AMI building is within 2 miles of the hospital ER where I worked. We began receiving AMI employees, postal workers, and community members who were frightened that they had been exposed to anthrax. They were also angry about the delays in treatment by public health. They wanted to be decontaminated, "checked out," swabbed and given antibiotics.

We had to triage those at risk from people with irrational requests. For example, one of the people interviewed was loudly demanding Cipro, yelling, "I've been exposed!" When asked why she was so concerned, her response was, "I drove past the building!"

We ended up sending 161 legitimate swabs to our lab. None of these turned up as positive for the bacteria.

Cipro ended up having to be rationed as people were demanding it inappropriately. There were people who flocked to their personal doctors demanding an antibiotic and then just hoarded it in their homes in case they began to feel ill.

Within weeks, Palm Beach County was not the only site of contaminated letters. Additional cases were identified in New York City, Washington D.C., and Connecticut. A total of 22 victims were identified, 5 of whom died.

Chlorine Dioxide was used to fumigate the AMI building. It remained sealed until the FBI closed their investigation in 2010. Eventually, the property was sold for $40,000 despite having been previously assessed at $12-15 million dollars.

The concern by the health department and fire-rescue were concerned that the pressure from the gas used could possibly have leaked spores into the surrounding environment from aging window seals. Rodents could possibly have been subsequently infected. Anthrax spores can survive for decades or even centuries. Disturbed grave sites of infected animals have been known to cause infections even after 70 years. This information was not disclosed to the public.

It was not until August 2008 that the U.S. Department of Justice stated that they believed Bruce Ivins, a senior biodefense researcher employed by the U.S. Government, was responsible.

There were many lessons learned from that incident in our community and nationwide. Improvements were made in hazmat protocols and equipment, risk communication, surveillance, mass dispensing of medications, and training for medical professionals. It inspired me and many others to be vigilant.

One of the themes of 9/11 is "Never forget". I won't.

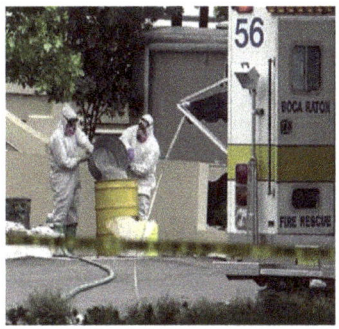

Puckered

In the ER, we would receive ambulance patients, usually of the frail, anxious elderly variety, with suitcases perched on top of them. They had nothing associated with an acute illness or injury but wanted to "check-in" as if the hospital were a hotel. That behavior became known as the "suitcase sign," and we saw it repeatedly with hurricanes despite lots of messaging to our physicians and the public.

In 2003, when SARS, also known as Severe Acute Respiratory Syndrome, was on the news, we received a rescue of a woman visiting with her family from China. They were staying at a large local resort hotel when she began developing a fever accompanied by respiratory distress. My staff were anxious even though they were geared up in PPE, and the patient was immediately placed in a negative pressure isolation room.

Not even five minutes after she arrived, I received a frantic call from the hotel manager asking what to do with the two thousand guests and staff who might have been exposed to what she had. Like we would know that quickly? Thankfully, it wasn't anything to be concerned with. But anxiety recurred when H1N1, a potential virus for pandemic influenza, arrived, as well as MERS, the Middle East Respiratory Syndrome.

The 2003-2004 influenza season was particularly bad. The media didn't help with reports of a "Killer Flu" affecting children in Colorado and then reported cases affecting both children and adults nationwide. Florida becomes a petri dish in the winter as seasonal 'snowbirds' and tourists flock to the warmer climate and transport their germs as well as their luggage with them. One night shift during the peak of an outbreak, our ER got overwhelmed. We were completely full- all beds, the hallways, the waiting room, and even outside the ER doors. People were frantic, banging on the triage door to the point where the door broke. I had to call maintenance and security to manage the situation.

The fear factor spiked again with news of the arrival of ill U.S. healthcare staff returning from West Africa and acquiring Ebola cases in two nurses in Texas in 2014. For healthcare staff, this initiated the need to know how to care for "suspect patients." There was frantic development of plans to receive such cases and the need to do our best to remain calm.

Training ramped up to a high-intensity level with the meticulous donning and doffing procedures associated with the type of personal protective equipment required, which labs to run and how to pack and ship them out, and a host of other concerns. There is always humor in crisis, and it became evident when I needed to scramble to find size 14 boots for one of my ER docs to be able to be dressed appropriately.

It didn't help to learn that we could be infected with a minute amount of the virus as these patients progressed to have projectile vomiting and diarrhea—liters of it. It is best practice to limit the number of personnel to care for such highly infectious patients, which means that nurses would do the cleanup. Lovely.

We could be quarantined for weeks after caring for a confirmed case. As an ER charge nurse, I also realized it was a staffing issue; I couldn't assign colleagues who were pregnant, had lupus or hypertension, or had young children at home who were dependent on them. The care and supervision needed to isolate and care for even one suspected patient were overwhelming. What would we do if there were many patients infected?

The pucker anal sphincter tightening factor emerged over and over. We had to manage concerns about dengue, Zika, Chikungunya, norovirus, etc. The media are counseled to avoid making false statements and inciting anxious viewers. The jury is still out as to how to inform the public without paralyzing them into inaction or frenzy. As healthcare staff, we will never stop worrying about the next mutation of an influenza virus, a mass shooting in our schools, or a severe weather event bringing us casualties. But we soldier on and huddle together to get through each and every one of these threats. We are the force to help combat fear among ourselves and others.

We could not have anticipated the scope and duration of the Covid-19 pandemic when it hit in 2020. It is one thing to care for one infected person. Quite another when it is hundreds and refrigerated trucks get parked outside hospitals to place fatalities. The morgue at my hospital can only hold seven bodies. The situation became a mass casualty incident on its own.

Falling

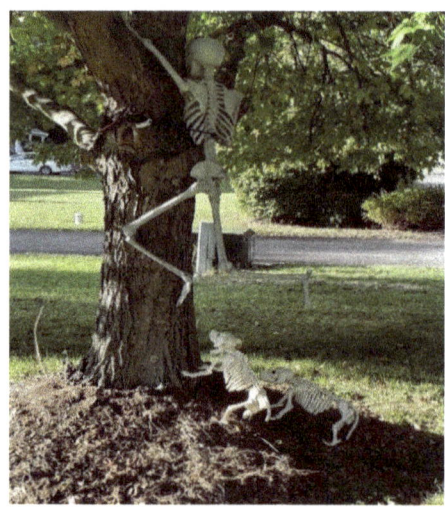

My younger sister, Norma, fell while attempting to bungee cord a Halloween decoration to a tree in her front yard- a skeleton chased by two small dog skeletons. She sprained an ankle but was otherwise okay. I told her I'd give her an award for a creative type of fall.

That got me thinking of the many varied stories of slip and falls, trip and falls, and falls from heights that I've seen as an ER nurse or know about from personal experiences. We have all fallen in our lives.

Babies fall a lot. They learn to sit up, stand, start taking a few steps, and then they progress to us running after them. Wearing a diaper helps in the beginning to cushion their falls when they plop down. They usually don't get hurt with all their falling unless they go forward and hit their heads. Or they get dropped accidentally.

Being closer to the ground helps a lot. The more adventurous kids get into trouble when they climb out of cribs, shopping carts, and strollers or tumble down stairs. We all know a child who has donned a mock cape around his shoulders, announces that they are

Superman, and proceeds to jump off beds, desks, and dressers. My daughter was convinced that she could fly if she believed it hard enough, like Peter Pan or, in her case, the tooth fairy.

Older kids get into more trouble. They fall off their bikes, swings, skateboards, roller skates. Most of the time, they sustain minor abrasions, small lacerations, bruising or maybe a fracture. Being young has its advantages- a cast is a pretty cool thing to show your friends, and you heal quickly.

It's a different story with teenagers and young adults. They tend to be very active and competitive. They play sports to win. Every sport has risks- gymnastics, football, hockey, basketball, track and field. Young boys think they are invincible. Getting hurt as a result of their actions is the farthest thing from their minds.

Friends dare them to do stupid moves like skateboarding on concrete barriers, ramps, and walls. Their falls tend to be associated with a higher level of injury, especially when they happen because of fights or things like falls from the beds of pickup trucks. Males tend to get hurt more than females. Getting intoxicated contributes to incidents like falling off sky-high heels for women, bar stools, or just plain passing out.

Working adults fall at their jobs- from ladders, roofs, construction site scaffolding. Sometimes, it is just a wet floor or going out when it is icy. There are always lots of falls with winter storms. It always feels like a shock to fall as an adult. Perhaps because we are taller than when we were babies- we have farther to go and we go down harder, so we break bones.

It doesn't take much for the elderly to fall. I took care of an older woman who fell and broke her hip when the wind blew her down. Another woman fell, trying to step on a cockroach that was trying to evade her. There are people who don't see those low concrete barriers in parking lots in the dark. Or they trip over their pets.

Then, there is a whole category of older people who have "fallen and can't get up." This can be devastating if they lay on the ground for hours or even days. Some of these are more memorable than others. An older woman in her late 70s fell while walking down her long driveway to her mailbox. Not only did she break her pelvis, but she sustained hundreds of fire ant bites covering her whole body before her neighbor spotted her.

Another case was a husband who collapsed and fell onto his wife, who was trying to break his fall. Both of them broke their hips. There was also a woman who lived alone and fell onto her tile floor in an air-conditioned house. She was not rescued right away, and her body temperature plummeted, lying on such a cold surface. In Florida, landlords have learned to do checks on elderly residents as some had been found three days later after storms hit.

A number of products have been suggested to prevent injuries from falls. Bubble wrap and small airbags that are placed over hips have been suggested but have failed to be practical. Wearing a diaper works for babies to soften their fall. Not so for adults. Hopefully, one day, there will be a better preventive strategy.

So, at least my sister had an interesting story to tell about her fall. We should all be so lucky!

Night of the Green People

Even though alcohol intake is frowned upon for those under age 21, it happens- a lot. Many adults view it as a rite of passage for young people that they need to learn their own tolerance and how to drink responsibly. Unfortunately, this is not always the case.

One of our three local universities decided to host a "Foam Party" to welcome new and current students back to campus on the first Saturday night of the academic year. It was advertised as an alcohol-free fun event with a locally known rock band. The recommendation was made to wear clothing that could get wet. In Florida, that translates to bathing suits.

The music started at 8 p.m., and initially, everything seemed to be going as planned. Participants were sprayed from head to toe with green foam. The guys were all shirtless, and they made sure that they were covered with the stuff—faces, ears, arms, legs, and torsos. The girls wore their bathing suits, too, and totally got into the frenzy.

Unfortunately, at the same time, clandestine drinking was occurring in the parking lots and dorms, unknown to the event planners. Word of mouth had apparently also spread to local high school students who had heard about this party and wanted to join in. They jumped the fences and infiltrated the mass of invited students, reveling in the spraying and drinking.

By 10:30 pm, things were totally out of control, with more than 1,000 young people congregating together, and there was trouble. The campus police were notified, and they, in turn, called local police for support to manage the crowd. EMS was called to assist with a large number of alcohol intoxicated and some injured students. They found unresponsive young people face down in the bushes and on the lawns. Many were vomiting. One was actively seizing. Some had fallen and sustained head injuries. A fight broke out in the melee, resulting in other injuries. There was also a report of a sexual assault.

Thankfully, the responders to the scene did their best. A police command vehicle was brought in. The music was halted, and an announcement was made for students to disperse and return to their dorms. A search began to locate those who needed care and transport them. The invasion of green people to our ER began.

They came on foot, by rescue, or crowded into pickup trucks or any vehicles that could be commandeered. It looked like a scene from a horror show on another planet.

My ER has fifty beds plus additional hallway spaces. It had already been a very active Saturday night, so the influx added to the drama. There were green ill and injured people in every available treatment space, as well as all the hallway stretchers. Many were actively throwing up on themselves and on the floor. A number were moaning; others were silent and unconscious. A few were laughing hysterically at the way everyone looked.

Our waiting room was filled with more green people-roommates and friends who accompanied those needing care awaiting evaluation and those who wanted to check on the welfare of those brought by ambulance.

Our older patients were wide-eyed and stared at this spectacle. One woman with dementia asked if Earth had been invaded by an alien species. Others just chuckled at the sight. Our ER staff just took it in stride as just another science fiction type of occurrence.

It did serve to be an interesting and memorable night. We were able to clear most of the green patients by 5 a.m. and all of them before day shift reported. The police assisted us with notifying parents of the high school kids to pick them up. Even the arriving parents were not expecting their children to look as they did. All of the minors were given a stern warning about their behavior and the legal age to be drinking, in addition to discharge instructions.

Follow-up phone calls were made to the university, and they have never had another Foam Party that I am aware of.

To this day, anyone who worked that Saturday shift still refers to what happened as the Night of the Green People.

A Close Call

The rescue call came into our ER as a 32-year-old security guard with dizziness and a headache. He looked pale and was holding his head but was able to communicate. When asked if there was anything unusual at his work site, he mentioned that there was "a lot of construction going on with hurricane damage repairs." Our next question was if there were any generators being used, and he nodded yes, but there were several.

A quick vital signs check using our new finger probe device to check for possible carbon monoxide exposure noted a markedly high reading. I asked if the building was occupied, and he said, "Yes, it's a 20-story condominium and fully occupied with mostly elderly residents". WHOA.

He immediately received a non-rebreather oxygen mask. I then ran to our "hot phone." It is a bright red phone that is part of our communications system located at our charge nurse station. It instantly connects to both police and fire dispatch when you pick up the handset- no dialing needed. It is a lifeline to request rapid assistance.

I relayed that we had received one patient with apparent carbon monoxide exposure and requested a hazmat team to check the building as there might be other affected occupants. Our ER has a great relationship with our first responders, and they immediately sent out a crew. Meanwhile, our security guard was already beginning to feel much better, and I moved on to assess other patients.

Carbon monoxide (CO) poisoning can masquerade with a multitude of symptoms, including nausea, vomiting, fatigue, weakness, headaches, impaired vision, a lack of coordination, chest pain, shortness of breath, and in really severe cases- loss of consciousness and death. The gas is odorless, colorless, and tasteless, so it can be undetected until too late. If you aren't always considering it as a threat, it can be easy to miss.

It is a leading cause of poisoning in the United States associated with fires, boilers, furnaces, vehicles, woodstoves and any combustion releasing equipment. Unfortunately, such poisoning is too common in Florida as generator usage has increased dramatically after some of our major storms.

In the past, our ER had received whole families poisoned when a generator was used inside their house. Typically, there is a lack of awareness about the risk; sometimes, it is simply to prevent stealing. It can also be due to an elderly person forgetting to turn their car off after parking in their garage or someone intentionally trying to commit suicide. We had even received patients who had lost power in their homes and left their windows open to get a breeze but became ill from fumes from the generator used by a neighbor. Usually, there are a limited number of people who become ill or die from such a cause.

On this particular day, a short while later, I was paged overhead back to the hot phone. The fire rescue lieutenant said that the carbon monoxide reading in the lobby of the building was 900 ppm (parts per million), 100 times higher than what can be considered normal and a potentially lethal dose. They immediately halted the generators, called for backup, and began clearing the structure. This included door- to- door searches to evacuate the mostly elderly residents- at least 100 of them in the building at the time. They began assessing all those evacuated for possible exposure.

We prepared for a potential surge of patients, alerting administration and our ER team. Rooms with admitted patients were cleared, and respiratory therapists were on standby. We remained on edge. A follow-up call about 15 minutes later came from the scene that only one other person was symptomatic with an elevated carbon monoxide reading and chest pain. He was transported to us at the ER. I was finally able to take a deep breath hearing that so many other unsuspecting people were not harmed.

When the building was further assessed, a discovery was made that an unlicensed sub-contractor team had inserted the exhaust from a large capacity generator into the ventilation system of the building. Another generator had also been running in the garage. Had the poisoning gone on any longer, it could have caused a mass casualty or a mass fatality incident for everyone in the building who inhaled the fumes.

What a tremendous relief that a tragedy was averted in time. I was grateful that our hospital had purchased rapid diagnostic point-of-care testing devices to avoid delays in detection. It used to be that you had to draw blood from an artery and run the test in a lab. Precious minutes do make a difference.

But the challenge remains. Prevention of carbon monoxide poisoning is an ongoing issue as it is now required in Florida that all nursing homes and other ambulatory healthcare facilities are compliant with having a generator. Supermarkets, gas stations, and big box stores have also installed them.

New homeowners of such equipment may not read the attached instructions and may also be delinquent in ensuring that there are available working CO and smoke detectors. Those who do not own a generator but open their windows to allow ventilation when their air conditioning is off can still become poisoned from a neighbor's fumes.

Most of the time in the ER, we make a difference for our patients, one at a time. Our motto is "We don't just save lives; we save lifetimes." Most of the time, it is a thankless job. We know how to provide necessary care for each person in crisis. But this is one of those instances where the outcome could have been altered for so many. It was a humble reminder to always think beyond what is in front of me. It could make a difference for others. This case opened my eyes to a public health perspective, allowing me to think beyond one patient at a time and to think bigger. Some say it's like seeing and thinking about things from a 10,000-feet-up approach.

Modern Day Nightingales

Florida is no stranger to storms. In September 2019, Hurricane Dorian approached Florida as a catastrophic storm, and the drill repeated itself. Everyone scurried to top off fuel, water, food, and batteries. The search to locate where the flashlights were around the house and if they were viable was completed. Patio furniture and anything that could blow away had been brought inside garages or homes. Those who have shutters put them up. Neighbors helped neighbors to prepare. The anxiety level escalated with the approach of the storm and the associated intensity level. People start stress-eating their hurricane snacks even before the power goes out.

Those who can evacuate do so. One of the unfortunate consequences of a storm is power outages beginning before landfall as the outer fringe bands come on shore. After a rainy, wet summer season, it doesn't take very much rain to cause flooding, especially on low-lying roads and properties. Normal temperatures are typically in the 90-degree range, but without air conditioning, the temperature inside homes and buildings rises to 100 degrees or more. It is too warm to sleep well or feel comfortable. Anxiety levels continue to rise, and people resort to alcohol intake. It is a staple hurricane supply for almost everyone. The number of domestic violence episodes increases.

As a child growing up in New York, I remember storms that came up that way and knocked out power and blew down trees. In Florida, it became a totally different experience over the course of the 35 years of living there. My first exposure occurred when Hurricane Andrew came ashore as a Category 5 storm in 1992. I was working ER in Palm Beach County and it felt like wartime even though the biggest impact area was south of us.

There was still enough local damage in Palm Beach County to cause lots of injuries. We went through cases of tetanus for those unlucky enough to get puncture wounds. The first patient that I cared for post-storm was a man who went up on his roof with a chainsaw to remove a tree that had fallen on his house. He ended up falling face-first off the roof onto the still-running chainsaw. That storm was the first time I heard of "chainsaw massacre days" with injuries rivaling any horror movie.

Our staff received patients by the busloads evacuated from hospitals and nursing homes from further south. Some long-term care residents had been evacuated to local shelters, but when the shelters collapsed. They were moved again to temporary locations like churches. I remember caring for elderly survivors who came to my hospital three days after the landfall of the storm. They all had that shell-shocked look.

Many nursing home residents arrived bearing water-logged, unreadable identification bracelets and without accompanying medical records. A number were in congestive heart failure after not having had their cardiac medications for an unknown period of time. Some had not had their diapers changed in three days. Family members began calling from all over the U.S., searching for their loved ones- fathers, mothers, sisters, brothers, and even children. Young children did get separated from their parents during the chaos of emergency evacuations. Great effort was taken to reunite families.

There has been a veritable alphabet soup of storms since Andrew, all with their unique characteristics. 2004 was a particular challenge as the names for our storms used up the entire alphabet, and the National Hurricane Center had to start using the Greek alphabet.

When you work in a hospital, there is a disaster clause in your employment contract that you will be available to work. Before the beginning of the annual hurricane season on June 1st, there is a mandatory signup posted in each department. You are given a choice either to work during a storm (Team A, also known as the Alpha team) or post-storm (Team B, or the Bravo team). I've had to work both teams as staff and as part of the Hospital Incident Management Team.

Those on Team A go into lockdown mode hours ahead of the anticipated arrival of the first big bands of wind and rain coming ashore. It looks like a giant sleepover as everyone starts coming at the assigned time, bearing their suitcases and pillows. Staff who have pets tend to sign up for post-storm shifts as they seek comfort from their pets and do their best to keep the animals calm as well.

Hurricane Wilma knocked out power to 82 hospitals in South Florida in October 2005. Even though my hospital had backup generators for critical life-safety equipment, there was only minimal lighting in many areas, including the stairwells, hallways, and patient bathrooms. The decision was made to move patients out of their rooms to the hallways to protect them from windows that could break with the high winds. And they did break- violently. Glass shattered all over some of the rooms, reaching to the doors going into the hallways.

The nurses used the modern equivalent of Florence Nightingale's lamp- flashlights and headlamps. I'd never really connected with the lamp as a symbol of nursing until I witnessed my colleagues moving in the dim light from patient to patient, offering words of comfort, checking temperatures, pulses, respirations, and blood pressures, and offering medicine to relieve pain, adjusting and repositioning pillows, bandages, and splints and basically doing the work of nursing.

Water penetrated aging window seals in the critical care units, creating unsafe conditions, so staff and patients were evacuated to the post-anesthesia care areas. This was no easy task as ICU patients tend to have IV poles adorned with lots of bags of medications and they need accompanying oxygen often delivered with manual bagging. Multiple staff are needed to move each ICU patient.

Buckets and barrels were placed in hallways to catch water trickling down from roof leaks. With reduced chiller support, the temperatures inside the hospital rose and everyone was sweating and uncomfortable. The walls and floors became slippery, too.

Staff were fearful about their family members being left in the care of others in their homes and in shelters. I remember personally comforting one of our security officers who broke down in tears and was concerned for her family. The hospital did allow a limited number of dependent family members to be brought to the hospital.

Everyone worried if their homes would be destroyed? Could they afford repairs? How bad was the storm really going to get? How long would lockdown last? During storms that stalled, it could last days. Those of us that had been through prior storms counseled our younger or newer coworkers on essentials to bring. Humor became a great coping strategy, and all sorts of comic commentary was circulated.

Typically, there is a surge of arriving patients before the big storms hit. Parents want their children checked for possible ear infections or respiratory ailments; there are lots of people with back pain from putting up shutters and getting hurt in the process. There were always frail people with their suitcases perched on top of them being transported by EMS and asking to be "checked in" because they were worried that their conditions would deteriorate if they stayed home and then couldn't get out. There are also community-living ventilator-dependent patients who seek safe harbor during the storm.

When the winds are sustained at tropical storm level, usually about 40 mph, the ambulances no longer can go on calls. However, that doesn't stop people from battling the wind and rain and coming to the ER in their own vehicles, although the volume is much lower. We got everything from gunshot wounds to women in advanced stages of labor, making it into us. There was even a police officer who had a deceased person sitting, strapped in by a seatbelt, in the front seat of his cruiser brought to us as he didn't know where else he could safely transport the person because of the high winds.

When the winds started to die down is when the surge of humanity really began. One of our local fire-rescue agencies notified us that they had 140 rescue calls that they had not been able to respond to that would soon be coming our way. As the only location with lights on because of our generators, we became a beacon for the community.

Our waiting rooms bulged so much that we ended up getting all the folding chairs out of our education center and making waiting areas outdoors. Our 'mammovan' turned into a minor care area for those who needed simple wound care and a tetanus shot. We lined up chairs in one of the hallways in front of treatment rooms for suturing. Stretchers lined every possible wall.

That first week after Wilma, we had treated 3100 patients. Staff were beyond exhaustion. When you got to finally go home, it was a frightening time to negotiate the intersections as none of the traffic lights were working. The roads were in total darkness and the flooding made it hard to determine how deep the roads or canals really were.

When we finally reached our home locations. There was, of course, no power. Yet there was much work to do to clear the downed vegetation, put a tarp over the new holes in the roof, mop up the floors where water had come in, and throw out all the decaying refrigerator items. The neighbors had all enjoyed a block party, cooking up their refrigerator and freezer items for everyone and talking about their own experiences. It was probably a good way to have a debriefing for them. I always missed those times because of lockdown.

When home at night on days off, it was so hard to sleep in the heat. The battery-powered fan I had wasn't powerful enough, nor did the batteries last long enough for a good night's sleep. We had to keep the windows and patio doors open for ventilation in the house. This, unfortunately, allowed the mosquitoes, palmetto bugs, and even snakes to get in. Noisy generators could be heard for months after storms. We treated whole families for carbon monoxide poisoning.

Florida has learned to prepare for higher levels with each successive storm. We look at it as reviews of what happened and what we would do differently the next time, calling it the good, the bad, and the ugly. Our state also helps other communities that get the brunt of these storms. We send search and rescue, disaster medical assistance teams, and lots of volunteers who bring supplies and services.

Hurricane season ends on November 30th each year. Thanksgiving is always a time to be grateful to have survived another year with family and friends. And then time to rest and recover.

Biobombers

For centuries, the military has acknowledged that you do not have to kill an enemy with violence. Disabling them is also an effective strategy. Documentation on the use of bioweapons dates back to the Bronze Age. Invaders drove infected victims into enemy lands, poisoned wells, dipped their spears into cadavers or excrement, threw infested bodies over walls, and deliberately caused outbreaks. There was no immunity from agents like smallpox or the plague. Even using a virulent transmissible biological agent via an animal or human or contaminating a food or water supply can be a covert way to wipe out an army camp or a society.

In our modern world, global travel has expedited the insertion of illness through travelers. Often, this is unintentional, but people do purposely ignore the risk of sharing their germs.

I remember caring for a man who presented to our ER in the middle of the night with intense vomiting and diarrhea. As dawn approached, he became extremely anxious to leave once he began feeling better after being given IV fluids and medications. He and his wife were so insistent that I asked him why he was in such a hurry. He would benefit from us monitoring him longer. He replied that they were booked for a cruise leaving that morning, and they did not want to miss it.

I offered to get him a travel note that he could give the cruise line to rebook travel for another date, but he refused. Despite repeated counseling by our ER doctor and me, he signed out AMA (Against Medical Advice), and I am sure he went on his cruise. At the time, it was not unusual to hear of outbreaks of norovirus on such vessels, probably from self-centered people like this person and unforgiving policies to refund travel cancellations due to illness.

After two years of our COVID-19 pandemic, people were anxious to travel again, mainly to warm locales during a cold, snowy winter. Not all airlines required vaccinations, and some were lax with mask policies. Testing could be unreliable, too.

People can thus become individual biobombers, causing illness to others. They can also sabotage infrastructure, causing significant disruptions.

I experienced this firsthand when, suddenly, the water in my hospital was deemed unsafe by our city water management. Apparently, a disgruntled, recently fired worker intentionally contaminated the system. He did this when we were receiving a surge of patients with norovirus from a nursing home.

I remember working at the bedside of an elderly woman who was just continuously erupting liquid stool out of her diaper, causing a river of feces to run off the stretcher onto the floor. It was a total mess, what we call a "Code Brown" in the ER.

You don't feel clean after such an incident despite wearing gloves and a gown. As I finally doffed my filthy gloves and went to wash my hands of any lingering infected material that might have splashed on my arms, I discovered there was no water to scrub with. It had been turned off.

Those cans of disposable wipes just don't cut it for certain circumstances. The police did identify the perpetrator, thankfully but it got me thinking.

We were used to putting on masks for the annual influenza season, but it made sense that maybe we needed to also think about pathogens from GI illnesses such as from C. Difficile or others. Did we need to wear even more PPE to protect ourselves from germs. Could our patients be biobombers without knowing it?

It's common for hospital staff to become ill from our patients. We do build up an immunity, however with being an international destination such as in South Florida, we get a number of different strains of each virus. Flu is notorious for having prevailing strains in addition to others which are not identified in time to include in vaccines. I think we all understand that now with Covid-19'variants.

I thought of the Charles Shultz character called Pigpen, a member of the Charlie Brown gang. He was always pictured as being surrounded by a cloud of particles because he was messy. What if our patients had an aura of invisible infectious particles that enveloped them that we could inhale and become sick from?

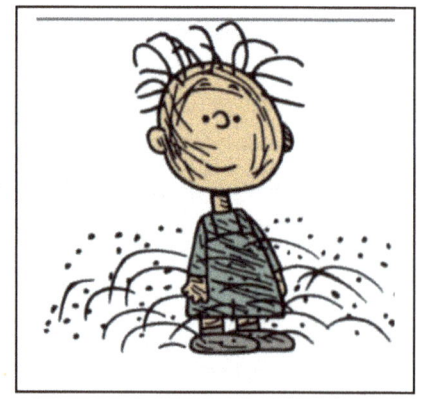

When people pass gas, those around them can detect the odor and hopefully escape it quickly. But working at the bedside trying to help someone in distress is not an option. It made sense to me that anyone with diarrhea could be potentially infectious to us.

I asked our 3M rep (PPE vendor) if we needed respiratory protection for our ill patients, such as those with vomiting and diarrhea. My query was posed to their research team, but it had never been specifically studied. I never got a good answer.

Any of us could potentially be a biobomber, right? Or be infected by one. Wow, that brings policies and a national strategy to a higher level across our society. I can only imagine how such thinking could increase paranoia and conspiracy theories, or maybe we will learn how to protect ourselves better.

My Chicken Disability

I'll admit it. I am the biggest chicken compared to anyone I know. Growing up, my sister Rita and I would watch "Chiller Theatre" on Friday nights. Our parents would often be out with friends or whatever it was that they did. We would sit next to each other in the dark on the den couch.

Every episode was terrifying, but we endured it even though most of the time, I covered my eyes with a shoebox. Each show would always start the same way, with a decrepit, gnarly looking hand coming up out of the ground and descending back to earth as the words "Chiller Theatre" resonated. I think I stopped watching it after one particular episode called "The Crawling Eye." The nightmares were just too much. It didn't faze my sister at all; maybe because she was a year older or, more likely, she was just braver.

I met my future husband while still in an undergraduate program. He learned pretty quickly about my chicken disability. We went to see the movie Jaws one night on a date and sat pretty far back in the theatre. Maybe it was the music "dun dun dun dun dun dun dun dun" which built up the suspense for the great white shark to appear out of the deep and attack an unsuspecting swimmer. All

I know is that I screamed so loud when it did surge out of the water that I made everyone in the whole movie theatre jump. I made that movie feel very real for everyone. Of course, everyone turned around and looked to see who screamed so loudly. I was a bit embarrassed but really, really could not have avoided doing that. My soon-to-be husband slumped down in his seat, but he still said that he loved me anyway.

Watching the first Jurassic Park movie was no better. I like dinosaurs, and the idea of a theme park centered around such prehistoric creatures sounded really good. I did okay up until the water started shaking in the glass on the dashboard of the car in which the children were riding. There was that anticipation again. Uh oh.

Then, the T-Rex appeared with its monstrous head and ugly teeth and chomped up the poor guy trying to hide in the toilet. Of course, I screamed. My three young nieces with me laughed at my reaction. It went downhill from there. By the time the raptors started jumping out and attacking people, I was past being traumatized. My nieces never let me forget that experience. I decided against watching future versions of that movie.

Early in my nursing career, I worked at the V.A. Medical Center in East Orange, New Jersey. I thought that some of my experiences there would help my chicken heart, as I was in the presence of veterans who had proved their own bravery.

One day in the ICU, a hallucinating younger veteran jumped out of bed; he picked me up and attempted to throw me out a glass window four stories above the ground. It was a close call, but I survived that episode, too. You might think I would be cured of my chicken disability by working at the V.A., but not so. I was still afraid, but mostly only on the inside. I learned to control how I reacted, at least. I also learned to be brave. Maybe I could become a master chicken!

Having children does make you stronger. It is our job as parents to help them understand their world as they see it. My kids were pretty fearless, though, and did not exhibit the inheritance of my chicken gene. In fact, they capitalized on knowing that they could make me jump at a fake but realistic-looking snake or spider strategically placed for me to almost step on or sit on.

My daughter marvels at how I can work in hospitals and deal with the horrible things that happen to people and yet be so afraid. Probably because, at least most of the time, the ill or injured are not jumping out at me deliberately. I learned that trying to be as prepared as possible for anything that might come my way has helped. Education is a powerful defense tool as you can logically analyze things and respond appropriately. When you are busy responding, you don't have much time to think.

But I have definitely been afraid on a number of occasions working in the ER environment. People who have overdosed on bath salts or flacca are crazed out of their minds. I think that having some options to physically and chemically restrain them helps, as well as having other people around to gain control of such situations. These things have helped me to manage my inner chicken.

When you gain experience, you accept the need to lead others. That's the bravery counterpart of. I will accept the challenge of a really difficult, complex situation. So maybe I'm a chicken braveheart. I don't think that I will ever be cured. In the meantime, I'm happy enough to regulate what I watch on TV or in the movies. I love films made for young children. One of my favorite movies is Babe, which is about a pig on a farm.

My career no longer has an intense clinical component, either. So maybe I can hope to ease into an overall calmer environment and ease my chicken heart.

Night Predator

Night shift always started very busy, with all treatment rooms filled and a list of people registered but waiting to be seen. By two in the morning, it was usually more manageable, so we could start relieving each other for breaks. Inevitably, the pace would pick up again as the bars closed at five a.m. Drunks would crash on their way home, sometimes alone, into trees or ditches. Sometimes, they drove the wrong way on dark roads, hitting other unsuspecting cars. There were also very early morning persons who awoke with congestive heart failure or stroke symptoms.

It was always the luck of the draw with how the nights went. Some nights were crazy, even insane. Others were fairly routine. So much of what the ER staff saw on their night shifts was preventable, either because of alcohol, unfortunate decisions, or plain stupidity. With two universities in town, the staff was used to alcohol and drug overdoses, fights over boyfriends and girlfriends, and anxiety peaks associated with midterms and final exams.

A major highway, I-95, was also nearby, and there were nightly motor vehicle crashes on that road and nearby secondary roads. People got used to driving at a higher rate of speed on the interstate and just didn't sufficiently adjust their speed appropriately going through the suburban roads. Everyone thought that they were good drivers and didn't realize that they could possibly be impaired by drinking, legally prescribed medications or recreational drugs, sleep deprivation, or distractions from everything, including others in their vehicles, cellphones, and music. The list went on and on.

There is a tremendous variety of illnesses and injuries seen in all ER's, affecting all age groups. On some nights, though, it felt like every single person coming in was vomiting or had abdominal pain or fevers or respiratory distress. The mental health cases also seemed to come in clumps. The staff would always take notice of a full moon, which they felt explained some of the craziness. My ER was similar to others. It made for interesting night shifts, especially as the types of cases seen in the ER on night shift are often different than what came in during daytime hours.

There were cases that got blood moving in the ER staff. Coffee always helped, too. Freshly made coffee was always the best, but most everyone would drink what had been made hours before, even when it looked like mud. By the time daybreak came around, and the relief shift started coming in, there was grateful anticipation of going home to grab breakfast and fall into bed.

There is a closeness that develops when dealing with difficult and unusual cases and supporting each other through tough times. Over the course of our careers, everyone accumulated their own collection of war stories. There were a few nurses and ER techs who were military veterans. They compared the ER as similar to working in a war zone at times. Preparing for each shift included mentally gearing up for the night to come and all that would occur. We were our own MASH unit.

People recognized me if I had cared for them before, but I didn't always remember them clearly. Cases blurred together with the steady current of incoming ones. Even though staff cared for people individually, with over 50,000 people seen per year, it was easy to understand when recall was difficult, except for those patients that stood out for one reason or another. It was enough to just focus on one person at a time.

Staff used the term wedgies to describe those who fall at night when getting up to go to the bathroom from their beds. People would complain of feeling dizzy as they rushed to make it to the bathroom, not taking the time to dangle for a minute to adjust from sitting to standing, or still feeling the effects of too much to drink before bed. People often ended up wedged between the bed and their nightstand or, alternately, the toilet and the wall next to it. It was not unusual to see at least one or more persons, both male and female, usually elderly, with a fractured hip or head injury every night. But my ER had some cases that didn't make sense, and we had to think like detectives.

One night around 3:00 a.m., fire rescue transported an elderly woman from one of the numerous nursing homes with a suspected hip injury. It wasn't unusual for that kind of injury. Usually, it was from a fall. The woman's left leg had the typical external rotation and shortening of a possible fracture. I completed the triage assessment and ordered the X-rays that would confirm the diagnosis.

I've always trusted my 'antennae,' imaginary feelers extending from my head when something is off and alerts my concerns.

The nursing home staff gave no history of any injury, including a fall. It wasn't unusual to get an incomplete report or a report of an unwitnessed injury. The woman was ninety-six years old with dementia. Also, it's not unusual. She was unable to verbalize beyond moaning, most likely due to her disease or maybe a prior stroke. However, she was clearly not ambulatory as she had severe contractures of her hips and knees and was diapered for apparent incontinence.

The other issue was the frightened expression on the woman's face, especially her eyes, which had a distant look of terror. Her whole body remained agitated as I checked her pupils, listened to her heart, lungs, and bowel sounds, and checked the front and back of her for bruises or wounds. There was evidence of some recent bruising on her hips and arms.

I wondered if the staff had been rough with her handling, lifting her into bed from a wheelchair or turning her in bed. Had she just been so osteoporotic that rolling her for a diaper change caused the injury? I documented my assessment observations and got a verbal order for pain medication from the doctor and gave it before I sent her for x-rays. I witnessed the same agitation when others approached the woman, including the X-ray tech, the ER tech who started an IV and drew her labs, and the doctor. It was a look beyond being in pain. It looked like she was afraid of something.

Due to a fever of 100.2, the ER MD ordered a straight-cath urine to rule out urosepsis. Because the woman would be unable to give a clean-catch urine sitting on a commode or the toilet, it would be necessary to insert a small plastic catheter into her bladder to retrieve a specimen. This would then be sent for a urinalysis and a urine culture. The catheter was immediately removed after the urine specimen was recovered. Having contractures and, therefore, limited mobility, it would most likely be uncomfortable to have the woman get into the frog leg position needed for access to her perineal area. With help from a female ER tech, however, we were successful in removing the woman's diaper.

I was as gentle as I could be, explaining what I was doing. The woman remained noticeably agitated during the procedure. I was glad that I had administered pain medication prior to moving her. She did have a heavy whitish vaginal discharge, and without a second thought, I swabbed it for a culture and then went through the procedure to obtain the urine specimen. Her urine was cloudy and a dark yellow color. Perhaps the woman had a urinary tract infection and was dehydrated, both common issues with elderly institutionalized patients. I informed the ER doctor of what I noted, and a culture of both the swab and the urine was ordered.

No surprise, the woman's x-rays clearly demonstrated a hip fracture, and she was admitted to Orthopedics for surgery to be scheduled for later in the day after medical clearance had occurred. After completing the initial admission orders, I reported to the inpatient nursing staff and sent the woman to her room. By then, my zone had two new patients to assess and care for in addition to needing to help with a cardiac arrest that a coworker was dealing with. I didn't think about my patient with the hip fracture after she left our department.

The following night, a rescue call came in at four a.m. announcing the pending arrival of another nursing home resident for a possible hip injury. I was the next up for a patient, so I ensured the room was ready. The woman was ninety-three and non-verbal, with a history of dementia. Again, no mechanism of injury was reported by the nursing home staff. It was a different nursing home from the night before. A phone call to the facility staff only yielded the addition that it was an unwitnessed potential injury. There were over 20 nursing homes in our hospital's catchment area, so receiving nursing home patients was a common occurrence.

EMS had found an older woman in her bed. She was diapered and had contractures on her arms and legs. Unfortunately, her x-rays were positive for a hip fracture, so I began initiating the admission and pre-op protocol for her. Another patient had another hip fracture. One more person in the incoming stream of those needing care.

After a busy night, I was grateful to have the next two nights off. I did my best to compartmentalize work-from-home life. I had to play catch-up with washing, bills, cleaning our home, making sure my children did what they needed for school assignments, checking on my aging parents, and hitting the gym. All too soon, it was time to go to work again.

As the staff in the ER break room began congregating to clock in for another shift at seven pm, I overheard another nurse complaining about poor communication and reporting from nursing home staff sending their patients to the hospital. I agreed with her. It was such a common problem. I asked which facilities were the problem that she noticed most recently. She told me the names of two familiar ones. I then asked, "Was there was anything unusual about those two locations?"

"Yes! They never seem to know what is happening with their residents. For example, last night, I took care of a woman with a hip fracture, but it wasn't clear how on earth it happened. The woman only moaned. That doesn't help me to figure out how her injury might have occurred. And the bizarre thing was that she was bedridden, so unless someone dropped her while transferring her from a wheelchair to bed, I don't understand how she broke her hip or when it actually happened. At 3:30 in the morning? And there was another one two weeks ago just like that."

It was time to get moving already, and I told myself that this needed to be documented and investigated. Were the staff being rough with their patients? Did they not know how to transfer frail persons or treat them with care? My ER had a process with a special form that could be filled out and put in my director's mailbox to alert her of a possible situation that warranted attention. It was inexcusable that cruelty might be occurring. I thought of my own parents and vowed not to have them placed in institutional care if possible.

That night was another busy one. A multi-vehicle pileup with three cars involved and 4 ambulance transports from that scene, 2 heroin overdoses, a psychiatric evaluation case, someone presenting with stroke symptoms, and several patients with chest pain, two of which needed immediate cath-lab intervention.

There was no lull from the incoming. It was a non-stop night. Early in the morning, another rescue arrived with an elderly female from one of the 'problem' nursing homes with a likely hip fracture. The similarity to the other cases I knew about was striking.

After taking the report from the EMS crew on this latest case, I was called to speak with a nurse on the 6th-floor orthopedic unit.

"We just had culture results come back from a patient you took care of a couple of nights ago. It is troubling because of her age. She is now post-op for a hip fracture. I am calling you though because her vaginal culture results that you had sent off are reporting that she has gonorrhea. I flagged her chart so her doctor will order medication to treat it, but I'm glad that you are working tonight to let you know as well. Something isn't right about it. She's from a nursing home and is bedridden. I can't imagine that she is sexually active."

I told her that we needed to follow up on the case, report it to her doctor and our supervisors, and notify the police to investigate it further. I was now worried our 'odd' hip fracture cases were possibly part of a series of occurrences. Were the two nursing homes linked in some way? Was there really some sicko out there who wanted to rape older women who were helpless and diapered? To do it, he must have used enough force to push their legs apart, causing their hips to break. And then possibly gave them an infection as well?

An Officer from our local Police Department took my call, listened intently, and said that he would stop by the hospital to speak with us further. He arrived 15minutes later. By that time, I was able to get temporary coverage for my coworker who had also expressed a concern so we could inform the officer about what we both had witnessed and our concerns.

The cases did sound similar. The officer asked us to generate a listing of the recent suspect cases that we could recall. Neither of us could immediately remember the names of any of the three cases we suspected. However, there was a way to do a computer search at the log for the nights we both worked. How many more might there have been? Hip fractures are seen frequently in the ER. The thought was frightening. The incidental STD result just added to the mystery. Was there a serial rapist on the loose?

All of the women were over 90 years old; all had severe cognitive and medical issues such that they required 24-hour care. None of them could walk on their own. All of them could not speak clearly, and all had sustained hip fractures. I also described the agitation I noticed associated with both cases that I was involved with. The officer left to speak with a detective from his station, and we both went back to take care of patients.

Before the ER doctor came to examine our latest hip fracture arrival, I alerted him to the possibility that the woman might also have been sexually assaulted based on recent cases and the culture result from one of the women.

No surprise, the x-ray results came back positive for a fracture. The police were still in the ER area, and I sought them out to let them know of a potential new case and a suspicion that there might have been a sexual assault. That would mean a rape exam.

I had assisted with rapes in the past but never on a person who was so old and frail. Together with a female ER tech, we anticipated that the woman would not be able to hold her legs steady to be examined. This patient was clearly upset as well. It was not an easy task at all to get the woman into a pelvic exam position and to endure the tedious collection of required specimens- swabs from every orifice, pubic and head hairs, nail clippings, and so on. There was evidence of trauma to her perineal area. Some bruising and bleeding from a vaginal tear.

The patient's gown and diaper were placed into evidence collection- the adult diaper being a first for me to turn in. Usually, it's just underwear. There is a strict procedure to ensure a chain of custody for evidence, and I made sure that we did it correctly. Besides the rape kit, She also sent off swabs to the tour lab for culture in case the woman might need treatment for a sexually transmitted infection. Cultures can take 48-72 hours to confirm an infection, so prophylactic medication was ordered. The entire rape kit contents were given to the police officer.

Then, I had to get the woman admitted so her hip could be repaired. After processing the orders from the orthopedic surgeon on call, I reported to the inpatient unit. My adrenaline level was still buzzing even though I was exhausted at the end of my shift. My eyes felt like they were burning.

It was a disturbing possibility to think about. The patient's chart indicated that she had been widowed. When was the last time that she had intercourse with her husband or anyone else? Most likely, it would have been painful for her due to her age, a likely lack of recent experience, and a loss of flexibility for sexual activity. If a rape had occurred, it could have caused the fracture in her hip.

I couldn't leave until an incident report on the suspect cases was completed and my nurse manager, director, and nursing supervisor were informed. Luckily, they all came in early that morning so I could get them updated on the situation in person and leave the next steps to them.

The investigation took on a life of its own from there. My director and my coworker told me that the police needed to formally get a statement from us to provide details about the cases that we were most recently aware of. The police had already requested staffing logs from both nursing homes on the nights in question.

In the meantime, the hospital's risk manager got involved and assisted with the notification to the next of kin of the need to treat the gonorrhea of the post-up patient. The patient's daughter was in her late sixties and was stunned by the news not only about how her mom most likely suffered a fractured hip but also of the STD that she would need treatment for. I was grateful that I did not have to make that call.

The daughter immediately wanted to remove her mother from the nursing home she had been in. She also wanted to press charges against the person who had done this to her mom once he was identified. Thankfully, her mom would first go to a rehabilitation center after discharge. The case manager would assist in finding an alternate placement for her. The officers could not yet tell the daughter that another nursing home was also suspected of other cases.

It didn't take long for the police to compare the names of staff at both nursing homes for the nights in question and to identify one male nursing aide as their suspect. He worked at both facilities on the nights that we had received the women with hip fractures. Healthcare staff often work a second job to supplement their income. He was brought into the police station for questioning as a person of interest in the case. He arrived still in his uniform from the shift that night.

The man vehemently denied committing any sexual acts with any of the residents. The police fingerprinted him and obtained an oral DNA swab. It was doubtful that any of the women would be able to identify him, but they photographed him just in case one of them might recognize him as an assailant.

Meanwhile, the police spoke with the directors of both of the nursing homes. They expressed genuine surprise that their employee might be a criminal. The director from one of the nursing homes said the aide had worked at their facility for 4 months already. She checked in with human resources department and they had validated his training certification. He had not listed any other facilities on his application as having worked at prior theirs.

The director from the other nursing home was very anxious but cooperative during her interview. She was totally unaware of any irregularities or issues with the suspect. Staff who worked shifts with him denied being aware of any of their residents being harmed under his care. Both directors agreed that during the investigation, he would be placed on administrative leave until there was confirmation of evidence that he might have been involved with their cases.

I was not included in further conversations about the incidents. I was just told that it was being investigated and that a person of interest had been identified. In the meantime, however, I was counseled not to speak about the cases as it could evolve into a potential public relations nightmare. I did read the daily local newspaper, but there was never any mention of what had occurred. Sometimes it can take years for cases to be processed.

When I later asked my director again for an update on the case, she told me that the man they suspected and then confirmed to be the rapist had been reported to the state board and fired from both institutions. To this day, I believe that it was just hushed up and not released as a story to the media. They would have had a field day with it. Vulnerable people who couldn't defend themselves against such a predator. Had there been other cases by him or others like his? Would there be others in the future?

Walk Slow

Some people have favorite phrases that they use frequently in conversation. One of these has stuck with me over time and has proven valuable in its simplicity and applicability.

I met Dr. Bob when I was working as an ER nurse. He was a crash reconstructionist- an engineer who analyzed vehicle crashes. It was a chance encounter that connected us.

Both of us happened to be involved tangentially with the same incident. An ugly one- a high-speed drunk driving crash at 2 am involving a sports car with four people inside wrapping itself around a concrete pole with tremendous force. Fire-rescue told us about "the eyeballs on the ceiling" of the car, which was particularly upsetting. All four occupants perished.

I just happened to be working in the ER that night and heard about the crash on our scanner. None of the victims were transported to our ER, however. They had been pronounced at the site, having unsurvivable injuries. We learned more from the traumatized firefighters who worked on the scene, who had to continue working afterward, responding to other 9-1-1 calls.

Dr. Bob was involved in the aftermath to determine how fast the car was going and any evasive maneuvering that may have been undertaken by the driver. He had been trained to look for skid marks, road, and weather conditions, and the forces upon impact.

Such high-profile cases often went to trial, and required impounding of the vehicle and methodical analysis in addition to law enforcement and fire-rescue documentation.

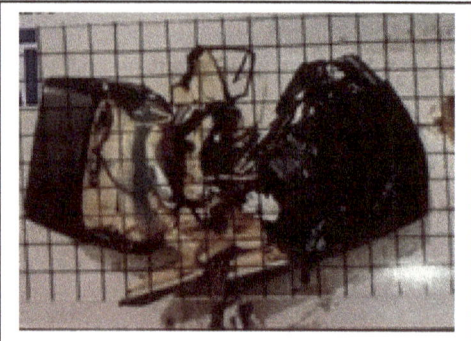

It was a lengthy ordeal and one of the vehicle photos wound up on Dr. Bob's business card.

I was always focused on the damage done to a person's body and could usually anticipate the injuries based on whether they used seatbelts, what they came into contact with, how the crash forces impacted their body, and if they had been drinking or speeding. This detective work helped with pedestrian vs. vehicle cases in addition to the roadway occurrences.

Occasionally, we would see tread marks if they were hit or ejected and then run over by another car, glass fragments, and vehicle paint chips on their clothes. The police have dedicated staff who take photos for evidence purposes.

Dr. Bob had a different perspective. His job was to figure out the impact of the crash on the person's car and the factors contributing to it. Often multiple vehicles were involved, so there had to be an analysis of the entire scene.

I found it fascinating that he focused on a dent in the dashboard or hair remaining on a spidered windshield, while I immediately worried about a head injury on the person who caused such damage.

Both of us used specialized equipment to do our jobs. For me, it was physical assessment skills, coupled with monitoring equipment, x-rays and CT scans, labs, and history that we could get from fire-rescue, other vehicle occupants, or police. He used survey equipment, gridlines, specialized software programs, and focused photo shots of various parts of the vehicle.

Fire-rescue would sometimes give us a Polaroid of a crash scene with the involved vehicles so we could see the type of impacts that had occurred. We looked for compartment intrusion, crush, and whether the airbags had deployed, and other such things.

Having a photo was often not an option as I worked night shifts, and many of the crashes happened late at night. It was usually too dark to get a good photo. For those patients who came in with a photo, it wound up as part of their medical record.

We knew that the city's bars closed at 2 am, which was often when the first wave of smashups occurred. Some people crashed even before they left the parking lot. The next wave was worse, after 5 am, when the bars in the unincorporated area shut down. Blood alcohols were especially elevated after hours of drinking.

Those crashes could be single cars going off the road into buildings, trees, down into ditches, or into canals. The occupants were often severely injured, and possibly undiscovered until daylight when there were observers to find them.

If the drivers were reckless enough to get on the highways, the result could be multi-car wrecks or wrong-way crashes. The latter were especially devastating as they usually involved a frontal or head-on impact with other vehicles at high speeds.

Every crash was unique for both occupants and the vehicles involved, so there was always a need to determine what exactly happened.

Dr. Bob had a lot more time at the scene than I did at the bedside. In my world, every minute counts with a major trauma patient. You had to think quickly and anticipate what to do, usually without help from the injured person. They were often unconscious, just moaning or shivering so badly they couldn't speak. We would do our best to stabilize them before transporting them to the OR or ICU.

Dr. Bob's mantra was "walk slow". He applied this to his work and to life's complexities. He taught me to not jump to conclusions, but to take a step back and let the evidence speak for itself. My timeline was just more accelerated than his.

Some use the phrase "let the dust settle" and it is close in its meaning to his phrase. I never got to ask Dr. Bob where he coined the term. I knew that he had been in the military, specifically the Vietnam War. Maybe that is where it came from, to avoid stepping on landmines? Or maybe from his experience as an industrial engineer before he went into crash reconstruction?

A systematic and disciplined "walk slow" approach was a good one for me to emulate. It worked for later research endeavors as well as when raising children, particularly teenagers. It meant being careful about making assumptions and waiting before you might say something in haste. It worked in everyday conversations. Not to be the motor mouth or the one with "verbal diarrhea," but to take a slower, more measured approach and think before you say something you might regret later.

"Walk slow" has another meaning for me as I am aging. I am less likely to trip and fall if I move a tad slower. Taking more time allows me to not only spot hazards but see details that I otherwise might have missed. It is easier to be a good observer if you take your time.

Walk slow is a good enough phrase to share with others, but I always think of him when I use it.

White Space

We were notified of an impending rescue call early one evening ER shift. A middle-aged female with a gunshot wound to her head. I had an available trauma room, and that night, I had a student nurse shadowing me.

I had warned her before we began working together that I could not predict what she might see as every night was unique.

Upon their arrival, fire rescue and the police provided more information about our patient. The woman had been found sitting on her oceanside condo patio dressed in a floor-length formal gown. It appeared to those present that she was watching the sunset on a beautiful night.

A gun was found on the floor next to her chair amidst a pool of blood. On the table in front of her was a glass of wine and a suicide note. Neighbors had called 9-1-1 after hearing a shot fired in their building.

She was in bad shape, apparently having chosen to insert the gun into her open mouth and fire. The police had already paper-bagged her hands to preserve fingerprint and gun residue evidence. They brought the suicide note in with them to be included in her medical record.

It was obvious that she was dying. She was unresponsive, and her respirations were agonal. The damage done was extreme in her mouth, causing serious hemorrhaging, and she had a large exit wound at the back of her head.

Chunks of brain tissue could be seen falling out of the temporary bandaging. The damage to her brainstem was irreversible, and she died within minutes of arrival.

It was shocking for a student to witness, but she was tough enough to handle it. We did post-mortem care together, and that was when she asked me:

Who cleans up the scene after a suicide or homicide?

I had never thought about it before but assumed that such a task was left to the criminal who might want to cover their tracks, those who knew the victim, or maybe an owner or landlord. We both hoped that it wouldn't have been her family to deal with the mess.

We asked the police officer who was present and was surprised to learn that there are dedicated 24-hour rapid-response specialty clean-up cleanup service companies that handle such requests for homes, cars, and businesses.

It must be difficult to enter people's personal space and find things left just as if they were going on with their lives.

Such a call is typically made after first responders and the police have completed their investigations. Team members are trained to be compassionate and discrete. They earn OSHA certification to clean and disinfect biohazardous materials, including blood and bodily fluids, chemical residue from tear gas, and even sticky fingerprint dust.

Good-to-know information that I filed away in my head, hoping that I would never have to deal with such a gruesome event myself.

Much later, I heard about one such call for help, which made me appreciate this kind of service.

An attorney called a homicide clean-up company following a particularly horrific attack on a Thanksgiving holiday weekend. He wanted the clean-up team to just let him know the final cost; no initial approval was needed, and it was essentially as if they were given a "blank check" written to fill in.

In this case, it was a couple who had been viciously murdered in their home by an intruder. Multiple rooms of the house were involved- the master bedroom, bathroom, and kitchen areas had blood spatter on the windows, walls, floors, and every possible surface. Both victims had been brutally stabbed multiple times until they perished.

Two clean-up team members arrived in their unmarked vehicle to avoid attention from neighbors. They immediately went to work after donning white coveralls encasing them from head to toe, boots, gloves, and masks.

It was a bad scene, as there had obviously been a major struggle. Furniture was broken and knocked over; glass was littered over the carpet and floors, and blood was just everywhere, even having hit the ceiling.

The female member focused on the kitchen, sweeping up the debris on the floor and then scrubbing the surfaces of the appliances and the countertops.

Then she saw it- the day-planner of the murdered woman. It was laid open on the central island area, and that is when she stopped short. Every day was crammed full of meetings, appointments, and commitments that the woman had made. It didn't matter what all those things were. There was no time at all carved out for that poor person. It made an immediate impression on her to make "white space" in her own life, beyond work and needless craziness.

The story was printed in our newspaper, and I took it to heart. My own schedule was packed with work shifts, community service volunteering, and with all the school and after-school activities associated with raising my own children. I was too busy!

From that point on, making more white space became my new goal. I actually put that story into my family Christmas letter that year. I realized that I had never learned how to say 'no' when asked for help, always managing to fit requests in. The hard part was trying not to feel guilty about turndowns. Decongesting my busy schedule, it took quite a long time, but I consciously worked at it. Family time took priority over everything else.

A wise colleague once told me that strategic planning involves deciding what is important to continue doing and making a conscious decision to stop doing what is less important.

I was grateful that this valuable lesson had been shared. None of us know how much more time we have on this earth. Making white space for personal time can help us both decompress and even accomplish other goals in our lives. A simple but powerful phrase.

The Teddy Bear Man

"A hundred years from now it will not matter what my bank account was, the sort of house I lived in, or the kind of car I drove... but the world may be different because I was important in the life of a child." —Forest E. Witcraft

Kids get scared when they become ill or injured enough to require care in an emergency department. Mostly, it is related to a fear of the unknown. "What will they do to me?" "Will it hurt? "Will I have to get a shot?" "Will I be alone?" "Will I die?"

I could always see when they are trying their hardest to be brave. Their faces are pale, and their expressions are fearful. Tears lurk at the corners of their eyes. They cling tightly to their parents, burying their heads into the bodies of those holding them, looking away, closing their eyes, and clenching arms and legs.

Fear escalates from doctor visits for well-child checkups. There is always the threat of another vaccination in addition to poking and prodding. What could happen in a hospital?

We were lucky in my ER to have a special patron, Mr. P., who understood how children might feel in such an environment. We called him the Teddy Bear Man.

Very few of my colleagues ever saw him. I did meet him one day when he came to visit our department for a drop-off. He was elderly, with grey thinning hair, a stooped posture, and a slow gait using a cane. He was very soft-spoken and humble about why he was there.

He had lost his wife years before and lived alone. I could tell that he loved children, and his face would light up when we shared stories with him about how he helped us make a difference with our kids.

His single wish was to make sure we had stuffed animals, especially Teddy Bears, to give to children who needed our emergency care.

Hospitals were not the ones which came up with the idea. Police officers initiated a program in 1997, called the Teddy Bear Cops. The idea for the program evolved after a Midwest story was published that involved a state trooper who gave teddy bears to two young brothers who had just seen their little brother killed by a car.

Giving out teddy bears to traumatized children in crisis can help to stabilize and comfort them after other horrific incidents such as rape or witnessing domestic violence that results in murder.

Firefighters followed suit, offering the soft toys after fires. The program began with 100 boxes of teddy bears and was met with an overwhelmingly positive response from police and fire emergency responders who were able to comfort small children at various disaster scenes.

"While law enforcement can't take away the hurt of a child's trauma, providing a comforting teddy bear may provide some help, and it may also help open a dialogue between the child and officer," said Chick, one of the police officers.

Nearly half of American children experience at least one or more serious traumatic childhood experiences, according to a survey conducted by the National Survey of Children's Health (NSCH). With so many studies linking childhood trauma to violence, depression, suicide, alcohol, and drug abuse, the importance of protecting the well-being of children persists. The pandemic has highlighted this continued need.

Stories about teddy bears are often familiar to children, including Winnie the Pooh and Paddington. There are adults who have faithfully kept their own childhood teddy bears. Mr. P. decided that he would carve out his own legacy for our hospital. I never got to ask him about his own background. Was he a police officer or a firefighter in his younger days?

He would bring a large bag to our ER stuffed with an assortment of stuffed animals. The teddy bears came in a variety of color shades. All were small. All were soft. The eyes were sewn sturdily, appropriate for even the youngest of children.

Every so often, there were other animals too- lions, zebras, dogs, cats, even a hippopotamus. We had a special cabinet designated for this stash to be used at our discretion as nurses. His only request was to let him know when we needed a new supply.

Not all of my colleagues took advantage of this. Some simply forgot we had such a treasure available or ignored it. Unfortunately, there are healthcare workers who are afraid of taking care of children and avoid them whenever they can.

Maybe because I grew up in a large family, I was comfortable around little ones. I knew to be gentle and talk to them honestly, but in terms that they could understand. Hearing medical terms can feel like being in a foreign land. I've been there. I understood.

I loved searching for the perfect stuffed animal for each child who needed extra support. It was a wonderful thing to see their faces light up and relax. Here was something fun to focus on, to hug, to take away the tenseness of the moment. It was a surprise for both of us.

It helped for them to have something to hold onto when we needed to do assessments, start IV's, draw lab's, inject local anesthetics before suturing, or administer interventions like nebulizer treatments. Many children are curious about things that they haven't seen before. Parents became less anxious when the child calms down. With children, you are always caring for the family unit.

The teddy bears were also terrific for explaining procedures to children. We could demonstrate on the teddy bear first, and let the child demonstrate back to us that they understood. Placing an oxygen mask on the teddy bear first made it less scary for the child. An empty needleless syringe could substitute as a "play" shot, for example. We gave them Band-Aids or small gauze pads to place on their own 'patients.'

After a laceration repair or splinting of a fracture, I would make sure to duplicate what we accomplished on the teddy bear too. All of this helped allay the anxiety of it all. The teddy bears could accompany the child for x-rays or surgery. One of our orthopedic surgeons always took the time after a procedure to cast the teddy bear's extremity, so it matched the child's.

Sometimes, there are no words to ease the unknown. *A* young girl came to us with an excruciating headache and blurred vision. Her CT scan noted a high-grade glioma in her brain. It helped her to have something to hold on to when we dimmed the lights in her room to ease her discomfort. We couldn't 'fix' her diagnosis, only help her cope a bit.

Mr. P assured us that his legacy would continue. He told us that his son would assume the responsibility when he could no longer manage it. In a world that desperately needs heroes, Mr. P was one of mine. The Teddy Bear Man.

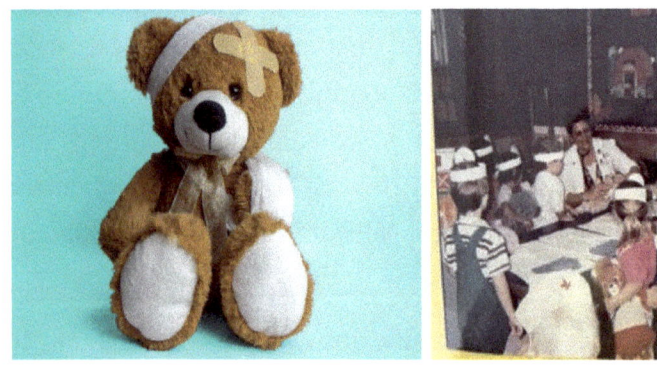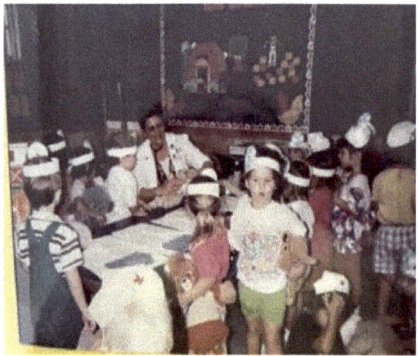

P.S. We took this concept a step further by offering "Teddy Bear Clinics" at our local schools. Children would bring in their own teddy bears (or favorite stuffed animals), and we would demonstrate how we would take care of them in the hospital. It was a great way to prepare them for not being afraid in case they ever needed us in an emergency.

Headlines and Bylines

Most trauma cases never become newsworthy. The media are most interested in those that are sensational and highlight people in crisis.

I have a binder that holds clippings of ER cases from my night shifts that did make the news that involved me as a nurse. This story is one of those, an early one from 1991.

The full scope of what happened in each case evolves in bits and pieces when more details become known. Usually, I would receive a quick summary of what to expect on the emergency radios, the arriving fire rescue and police officers, and then hopefully a first-person account from those injured.

I always got the "uh oh" gut feeling about an incoming rescue when the police crime scene technician would also show up in our trauma rooms. It meant that there would be more to the story being investigated, and it's bad. It also meant that documentation was critical as these kinds of incidents would progress to medical-legal court cases.

Clearly, our ER priority is always to stabilize the person and assess for injuries.

Just after 5 a.m., two young sisters arrived by rescue simultaneously after an assault had occurred in their home. The report we received was that one had a head injury, the other complained of ankle pain.

Both girls were traumatized, shaken, and sobbing. I was assigned to the older sister, Rose, 21 years old, with a head injury. She was barely coherent but was able to tell us what she knew while I was assessing her.

Her parents were "*always fighting*," and tonight did not seem different from so many others. The girls knew to retreat to their rooms when the yelling started. They just didn't want to hear all the noise, the shouting, things breaking. It could go on and on for hours.

Somehow, both of the girls were able to fall asleep. Then, early in the morning:

"My dad woke me up and asked me to check on mom. I wasn't fully awake but went into their bedroom. He was behind me. It was dark. She wasn't moving. Something was wet all over her head and the bed. Then my dad hit me with something on my head. Hard. Twice. Somehow, I ran away to my sister's room, woke her up quick, and we knocked out the window screen and crawled outside. I think he killed my mom."

One of the neighbors told police.

"I heard a woman screaming at her husband starting at about 4:30 a.m. I was half asleep, and it's not unusual to hear them yelling at each other about everything. They did it all the time."

Another neighbor called 911 after the girls ran next door to him for help.

"The one pounding on my door looked like someone had poured a pan of blood over her head. She was hysterical. The other one just laid on the sidewalk, all she was wearing was a T-shirt and panties. She was out of it."

Police recovered a bloody hammer at the scene that the father had used to bludgeon his wife. She was dead when fire rescue came. The father had apparently also used the hammer to hit his daughter. It explained her injuries.

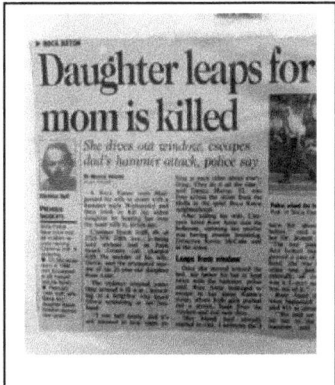

Rose's injuries were serious. She had deep scalp lacerations, still bleeding profusely, and we quickly learned that her skull was fractured in more than one place.

She was still processing that her father tried to kill her and might have also sought out her younger sister to kill her as well. Her actions saved both of their lives, but they had lost their mother, as the police later informed them.

The father fled the scene, apparently to go to his job on a

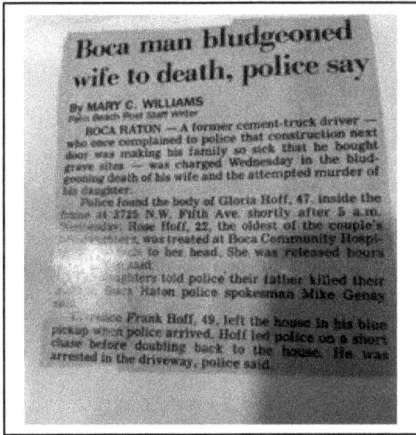

construction site. The police were able to take him into custody quickly, and he was transported to jail.

By the time I finished my shift at 7:30 a.m. and went home, there was no way that I could fall asleep. I was still absorbing the case.

Both sisters had been treated and were eventually released to other family members.

It was hard to fathom such evil. Thankfully, I had been sheltered from such violence growing up. I can only imagine that it would have affected me even more profoundly if I had been young and experienced such horror.

I was later served a deposition to relay my account of care for the sisters as the case went through legal proceedings. As is typical with so many ER cases, I did not learn how Rose and her sister did over time.

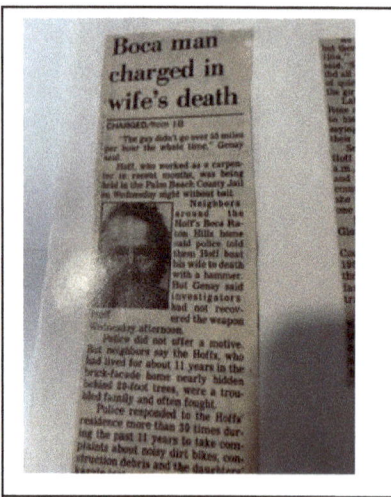

I can only hope that they both were able to survive their nightmares and eventually live in peace.

Another memorable case involved a 17-year-old teenager who came into our ER as a trauma case. His father got really angry at him when he hadn't taken out the trash when asked. His punishment was downright evil. The father locked him in a room with their pit bull and told the dog to "EAT HIM!". The kid survived but suffered dozens of bite wounds all over his body, including big chunks of flesh. The expression on his face was total shock. The police came and took photographs for a court case against the father.

I have never forgotten such cases. The pure evil still haunts me.

Rubberneckers

People are curious creatures, especially when there is the potential to see blood, gore, and human suffering.

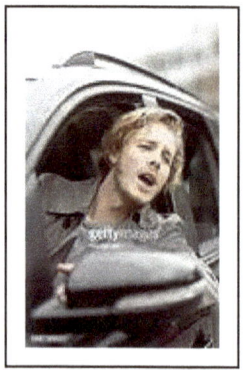

It's been like that for centuries, with paintings drawn and movies made during conflicts and sports events.

Gladiators in the Coliseum often fought to the death of their opponents, the audiences cheering as their favorites won over opponents. The drama intensified when the Romans added live animals into the arena to spice things up.

For me, this was a recurrent nightmare scenario, probably because I watched a movie depicting such scene. I made my dad always check that doors were locked to our home at night so the 'lions' wouldn't get in. It remains a mystery to me how I gained the courage to become an ER nurse.

Reporters look for sensational incidents, and in our modern world, their stories often include wrecks on the highways and roadways.

Bystanders and rubberneckers are commonplace, and what they see gets uploaded on cellphones or forwarded to media outlets. Traffic gets backed up every time there are police lights, "To see what is going on," "What happened?"

Wrecks can look awful, and those witnessing the aftermath wonder if the occupants survived. In the hospital, we would receive the injured, and we knew the answers.

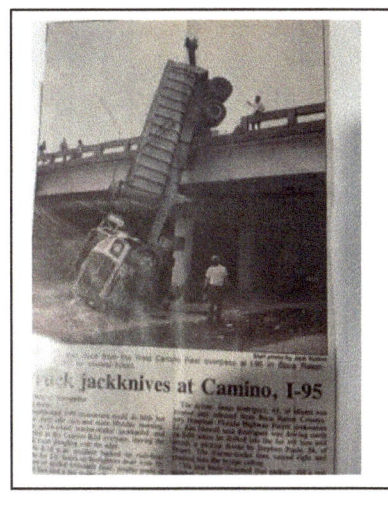

Truck jackknives at Camino, I-95

One of these crashes that made the paper happened at 6:10 a.m. on a Monday morning. The 43-year-old driver of a 14-wheel tractor-trailer lost control and smashed into a pickup truck on an I-95 overpass. The pickup truck was being crushed by the tractor trailer until released when the semi broke through the concrete barrier on the opposite side of the road and plunged to the ground below. The crash halted traffic for almost three hours as fire rescue extricated both drivers and managed both a fire in the cab of the tractor-trailer and a fuel spill.

I took care of the tractor-trailer driver who miraculously survived, only with a chest injury and bruises. The pickup driver escaped unscathed. I didn't see the photo of the crash scene until it was printed in the following day's newspaper. The pickup driver's car was completely totaled but was not visible in any of the published photos. As dramatic as the photo was, it proved that some of these incidents are survivable.

Others have not been as fortunate. I had just started a critical care night shift in the Surgical ICU of my hospital when we received a 32-year-old man involved in a three- car wreck. The story given to us was that he had run a red light exiting the I-95 off-ramp at a high rate of speed. His car hit two others, causing one of them to roll over. His vehicle then hit a concrete barrier, which stopped it.

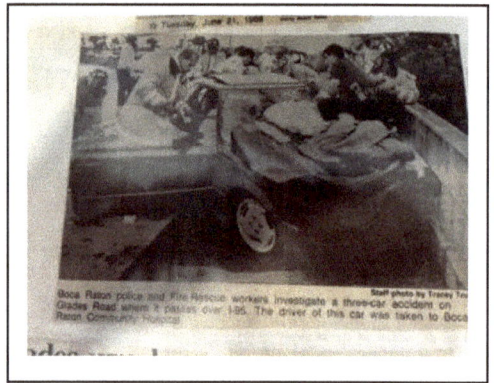

Boca Raton police and Fire Rescue workers investigate a three-car accident on Glades Road where it passes over I-95. The driver of this car was taken to Boca Raton Community Hospital.

He was unresponsive and sustained a major head injury. Because of the need to support his breathing, he was immediately intubated and placed on a ventilator. Externally, other than a few bruises, he looked okay. But his brain CT scan proved otherwise and reflected the result of transfer of high-energy forces. It would eventually be proved that he was brain dead.

He never woke up during the next eight days in our care. We came to know him after meeting his whole family- wife, parents, sister, and two brothers -during the short intervals that were allowed for visiting. As an executive of one of the local hospitals, his crash became another high-profile case. It was not an easy conversation to have with his wife about organ donation, but they were grateful for the option and approved it.

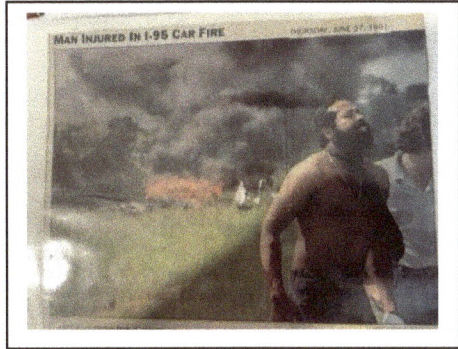

Bystanders can capture stunning images following some crashes. This 28-year-old man survived, although with serious burns.

There is always an unknown when police and fire responders arrive at a crash scene. How many people are injured? How bad are the injuries? How difficult will it be to extricate them?

Delays in care do make a difference. The need for the "Jaws of Life" is a red flag for more serious injuries, as people are trapped and time is precious to restore circulation to fractured extremities, to support breathing, and to decrease anxiety.

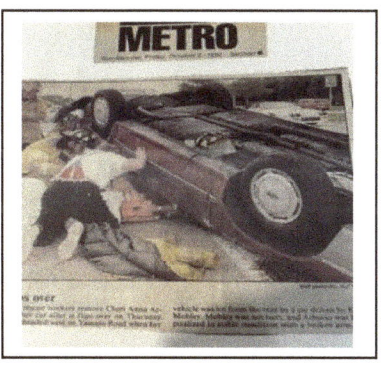

My binder of such cases is packed with clippings. They are all individual stories of which the outcome was not immediately known.

The bottom line is that all of these incidents become personal when you meet those involved, care for them, and do your best to ease their pain. I am thankful that I have the skills to be much more than a rubbernecker.

The Box in the Closet

It is awkward when parents talk about dying, but my mother was especially focused on it when she was barely middle-aged. Sometimes, she made threats to us as children when we caused trouble, saying, "You are going to make me have a stroke?" or "You will be the death of me!" She would also coerce my siblings and me to pay attention to what she wanted or maybe to evoke sympathy with a warning like "I can die at any time- the doctor said so!"

Such comments can be easily dismissed as an event that would not happen for years to come, especially when you are young, and your parents continue to survive. In a large family, we randomly took turns becoming the target for the death threats.

My parents did survive and were doing fairly well when they retired and moved to Florida into a house on the next street to mine. My husband and I and our kids got along with both of them. I was possibly the only one of my siblings that understood my parents and felt that I really was a true blend of the best of each of them.

I followed in my mother's footsteps as a nurse, and I know this did create an additional bond. She let me read her nursing schoolbooks, took me along when she did Red Cross disaster work, and, as I began my own nursing career, told me stories of her career as a maternity nurse, nursing supervisor, and educator. Needless to say, I was impressed with all that she had accomplished, and she also applauded my work.

I still heard my mom being fearful of death and wanting to be as prepared as possible. She even told my Dad that she intended to die first so she wouldn't have to be alone and miss him. She confessed that she did not want to deal with household finances and problems to solve. I laughed at this. Who gets to choose when they die?

Mom did some weird things like placing a piece of masking tape hidden on the back or the bottom of various things that she wanted to pass on to each of us children. We later found them behind paintings, under vases and cookie jars, in her doll collection, and knickknacks. When She asked us all what we might want in the house, I thought this was creepy and did not request anything. My sisters and brothers were more vocal, though. This led to a detailed inventory list that she wanted to pass on to each of us. But that was separate from the box in the closet.

One afternoon, my mom had me sit on the couch to discuss what she wanted after she died. Needless to say, I did not want to have such a conversation, but I knew that I had to listen to what she expressed. She said that after she passed away, I was to immediately go to her closet, find the box, and follow the instructions within. I agreed and just chalked this up to another of her strange thoughts.

I had helped her set up her closet when they first moved to Florida and knew that it was always organized—maybe excessively organized. She hung her clothes by season, purpose, and even color. She seemed surprised that I did not do the same in my closet. Anyway, I wasn't worried about looking for a Box in the closet if I needed to. In fact, I pretty much forgot about it.

The day came as a shock when I got a frantic call from my Dad to come over right away; my mom wasn't "right." When I got there, within minutes, I found out that she had been outdoors holding her beloved cat, Rosie, and it suddenly jumped out of her arms. She fell backward, hitting her head on the concrete pavers- so hard that their neighbor heard her fall. I knew this was bad immediately and called 911. She was transported to our local trauma center, and things happened pretty quickly afterward. And she did die.

133

My priority was to take care of my Dad. He was in shock over the whole incident. Then, I needed to call family members. Only after the arrival of my siblings did I even think of the box in the closet. No surprise, it was easy to locate. It was a simple box with my name and a large dried-out rubber band around it. Inside was a handwritten note on top of the tissue paper covering the contents.

"Mary- You are reading this as a result of my passing away. I have chosen you for a special task as I know that you will understand and honor this request."

She went on to tell me how much she appreciated me living near them and watching over them as they got older. And then came her specific instructions:

"I want to be remembered for my life in service as a nurse. Please dress me in my white uniform, stockings, and nursing cap. And don't forget my shoes...."

I cried when I read the note. It was so beautiful and perfect for how she wanted to be known. Of course, I did all of this in a loving way, as I completely understood her wishes.

Maybe one day, I'll designate my own Box in the Closet too.

The Limits of Hope

Hope is defined as wanting something to happen or to be true. I have personally struggled with having to be pragmatic and honest yet respecting how others desperately hold on to any shred of what they perceive as a positive sign.

I have witnessed the end of life many times in my career as a critical care and ER nurse. In both the ICU and ER settings, we would maintain a balance of respiratory support and a combination of intravenous medications to give every chance for a reversal of an impending death. We were bound to do no harm and offer every option to extend life; however, science and confirming diagnostics provided the evidence that what we did would likely be futile.

There is still a lack of understanding among many when efforts are failing, and hope dims. Family members want to hold on even when the bodies of their loved ones are weeping and necrosing. As caregivers, what we do to keep existence going is often painful-poking, prodding, disturbing what little peace and dignity may be left.

Family members want the truth yet to shrink away from finality-even in the face of such cases as a devastating intracranial bleed or when cancer is overtaking someone despite rounds and rounds of chemo, surgeries, radiation, bone marrow biopsies, failed stem cell transplants or other interventions.

I have borne witness to support the wishes of several family members who reached an endpoint for what could be done for them. The longer people live, the more we have come to know them and thus miss their presence. The difficulty is compounded when tragedy hits, and younger lives are jeopardized by illness or injury. We know that they had lived life with intensity, and the promise of what is still to come may be shadowed.

My family faced such an obstacle when my beautiful sister, Rita, bravely endured a battle with glioblastoma, the worst kind of brain cancer. Despite clinical trials and a seemingly endless optimistic attitude. The disease took its toll. She and her family were avid churchgoers with a strong sense of faith that with prayers, anything could be overcome. They could not see the loss of her abilities, even her awareness, diminishing.

I stayed with them at intervals to help. When I arrived for one of these visits, her husband, Kevin, insisted that I encourage her to use her walker more. They seemed surprised when I showed them how Rita could no longer use her left arm, and her left leg was too weak to support her. He grasped novel approaches to treatment that he read about, even though they were experimental.

Things went downhill quickly to where Rita became totally bedridden, sleeping most of the day; I had a painful late-night discussion with her husband about providing care and comfort to her at home with support from hospice. When I asked what was holding him back, what he said made me understand why he was resistant to accepting what was happening to her.

. *"I don't want to get in the way of a miracle".*

What could I say in response? I made sure that Rita had the home care that she needed, and it wasn't long before she passed away. Her family still seemed surprised that she could leave them. Over the years, I think about how people like Kevin hold on to endless hope. Maybe there are no limits to hope for them, or maybe they see hope as a lifeline to infinity instead?

Part Three
Pandemic Stories 2020-2022

Out of the Trenches. Still in the War. 7/15/2020

The Covid-19 pandemic has generated intense emotions and angst among all essential workers, particularly those in healthcare. Being close to those suffering from the highest viral loads places caregivers providing direct care at the highest risk. This has been a grim reality as it is estimated that 20% of such staff have been infected; some of these have died.

Even though I was now retired from working clinically in critical care and emergency departments, I felt intensely connected to what my colleagues who were still in the trenches were experiencing. Life and death settings created bonds from shared experiences. The staff I served with will remain my "work family." We were survivors together and continue to stay connected.

It has dawned on me that it may be like being in a war. The memories are enduring. Some are seared forever, not only into our brains but also our hearts and souls. Soldiers returning from conflicts do not share all they have witnessed with just anyone. There remains an endless processing of the sights, sounds, smells, and feelings associated with extreme incidents. Battle buddies are the ones who were there with them, who understand the moral injury, and who can relate to the complexity of recovery. I have served in my share of "wars," but this pandemic is beyond what any of us had gone through before.

Many refer to choosing a profession like nursing as a "calling," and they demonstrate a level of compassion and commitment to helping others, even under adverse conditions. Those who choose to serve in the military, work in law enforcement, emergency medical services, social work with the very young and the very old, and work within faith communities describe a similar revelation of the path they should follow for themselves.

In a pandemic, concern extends beyond worrying about personal safety, as in "Will I be exposed and infected?", "If I get infected, could I die?" to all those contacts beyond their work setting: "Will I infect my family?" "How can I continue to help my older parents?" "Who will provide for my family if something happens to me?"

Most of us have felt extremely vulnerable to contracting the virus. My brother, an attorney, told me about an urgent request he received from a respiratory therapist at a Westchester County, New York hospital early on in March for help in writing his will. This was a young person in his early thirties. They accomplished this task being on opposite sides of a glass door at the hospital where he worked. Needless to say, my brother was deeply affected.

What I do not yet fully understand is how there are so many people who feel that this pandemic is a hoax, a political ploy, or hyped as being worse than it really is. After thinking at length on this, I believe that they just do not know what we in healthcare do. They have not seen the struggles inside the emergency departments or intensive care units and the fear on the faces of those struggling to breathe without their loved ones near them. The fear of dying.

They do not see staff crying in their cars arriving at the parking lots at work, fearful that personal protective equipment will be there for them of the right kind that they don't have to reuse over and over. They know that they will be working to the limits of their endurance for thirteen hours straight or longer. There will not be enough breaks to hydrate or enjoy a meal. Their faces develop ulcers and rashes from the masks they wear tightly. They stay dehydrated so as not to have to remove their contaminated PPE to go to the bathroom.

Patients with COVID were medically complex. Many had underlying conditions to be managed. They usually required specialized airway support, such as high-flow nasal cannulas and ventilatory devices. Their lungs got obstructed from pneumonia and fibrosis, and they struggled to breathe even when heavily sedated. Turning them on their bellies to a prone position helped, but this necessitated lifting help to accomplish.

Turning someone is in excess of 250 pounds is not an easy task under normal circumstances, especially when they are completely unable to help themselves.

Because of visitor restrictions, the healthcare staff are the bridge between patients and their loved ones, beginning at the ER entrance and beyond. There have been many deaths from COVID-19, and this has been the toughest part of all of it. No one wanted the casualty count of this battle to be so high.

Staff were coming home from work to strip down their clothes and shoes, eat alone, and then sleep by themselves. They didn't want to bring the virus home, so they slept in their garages, basements, a work friend's house, or a hotel instead.

People were afraid to be associated with caregivers. So, they hid any evidence of their careers, changing into and out of uniforms at work so they did not get spit on and ridiculed. I worried about how much these caring people on the frontlines could endure before giving up.

Some stories were being told in the media, but were those who should be listening hearing them?

Endangered   11/25/2020

As the United States was in the throes of a third resurgence of the COVID-19 virus, the burden of supporting healthcare was evident in every state. Hospitals continued to complain of financial deficits; however, their current biggest concern was staffing. There had been a shortage for years, but now healthcare workers were on their way to becoming an endangered species.

It felt like we are now considered trophy animals to be slaughtered. Despite being recognized as unique and essential to our ecosystems, there was insufficient protection from threats.

Hospitals sought temporary contract employees to manage the exponential increase in those needing care without results. Everyone was vying for the same small, limited amount of available trained people.

Staffing ratios had expanded to near-crisis levels. Pressure was exerted on tired, overwhelmed workers to pick up longer or extra shifts. This had worked in the past, as people stepped up and helped out of a sense of duty and loyalty to coworkers.

For far too long, there has also been an extreme shortage of PPE- not the right level of protection, insufficient supply, poor quality items, and having to resort to conservation and reuse strategies that were national failures. As a result, one out of five healthcare workers exposed to patients with the highest viral loads had tested positive for the virus. Since testing supplies were limited, many staff did not know that they contracted COVID-19 until they became ill and wound up hospitalized.

The numbers of available workers were dwindling quickly without replacements. Fewer high school graduates expressed an interest in a healthcare clinical field. There were so many other choices that paid more and were much less dangerous.

Older workers were retiring sooner than they would have under normal circumstances. Pregnant staff feared for their babies and left the workplace. Increasingly, staff were voicing that they were so tired, burnt out from all the challenges, and totally frustrated with all the people who still refused to wear masks and follow social distancing guidelines.

"Why are we killing ourselves when clearly, there are still so many who aren't listening."

There was genuine concern about the lack of community welfare associated with protests, rallies, open and packed bars, and holiday gatherings. Yet, when many of these people became COVID-19-positive and ill, they felt entitled to demand the benefit of every possible resource despite their past behavior.

Sadly, Some healthcare workers shared their stories of family members who did not want them to come anywhere near them on Thanksgiving in 2020.

The general public did not fully grasp what it was like to care for COVID-19 patients. Because of privacy rules, those in COVID-19 ICUs were sequestered away from their families.

"I wish others could see what I see, walk in my shoes for one shift, and endure 12 hours of wearing a tight mask day after day instead of arguing about wearing a mask at all."

To become a competent paramedic, emergency or critical care nurse, respiratory therapist, or physician, one must undergo specialized training, obtain multiple certifications, and gain experience.

Currently, healthcare training programs are very limited in granting completion of studies without sufficient supervised clinical hours. The resupply lifeline for new workers is constrained, and no end is in sight. Healthcare workers are a finite resource.

This topic was exacerbated when my brother, Blaise, from Wisconsin, called and said, *"I've been exposed."*

He was one of two doctors in a 13-bed rural critical access hospital in the northwestern part of the state. Together, they managed the hospitalized patients, took calls in the emergency department, saw all the residents in the associated 50-bed nursing home, and ran the family practice clinics.

As was typical for others in rural areas, his hospital's resources were limited. There were no ICUs, critical care nurses, respiratory therapists, ventilators, high-flow nasal cannula devices, or advanced antiviral medications.

Blaise's partner had an acute knee injury and was scheduled for knee surgery the following week. So, he would be the sole available provider for the next month.

On a prior weekend, he was making rounds on admitted patients, including an 88-year-old woman with pneumonia who became critically ill. He was refused a transfer so that she could receive care at their larger referral hospital in Minnesota after being told that they did not have capacity.

His attempts to emergently stabilize her were unsuccessful, and she expired. When Blaise was finally able to review her chart, he looked to confirm that her Covid swab was negative. It was never done. The physician assistant who admitted her said that he did not want to swab her as she would need to be placed in isolation until the test result came back, and the hospital could not afford to expend that amount of PPE for her care.

It was definitely a failure of hospital policy, but the pervasive attitude at the hospital was that Covid was not a concern for the hospital and that masks were not even necessary to wear by staff.

My brother had butted heads with hospital administration for months to get a universal mask policy in place. He served as a physician representative on the Wisconsin Board of Health; however, they had been underfunded and understaffed for years. There was currently no county health officer. Blaise did his best to educate staff; however, there was tremendous resistance. The hospital administrator counseled him for being adamant about preventive measures. He modeled the way for them by wearing a mask, but no one wanted to listen despite the increasing community case counts. He even received an anonymous death threat.

Blaise insisted that the staff who cared for the woman and her husband be tested. They all tested positive. Blaise's first COVID test was negative, but he was awaiting the results of his second test to get out of quarantine. On day five, he still did not have results (another failure), but he remained asymptomatic, thankfully. He was wearing a mask.

If Blaise had become ill with COVID-19, no physician would have been at his hospital. Instead, the hospital said they would contract a telehealth hospitalist to provide remote guidance.

It doesn't take many staff members to be quarantined or become ill, which is a big hit for a small hospital that is already understaffed. Also, patients who are admitted to their hospital will need to sign a waiver consenting not to be intubated if a transfer to a larger hospital is unavailable.

It is said that bad outcomes often occur as a series in a chain of events. This is just one example of the need to nationally get our act together to protect our healthcare workers everywhere.

Are we endangered or going to become extinct?

Making it Personal   12/2/2020

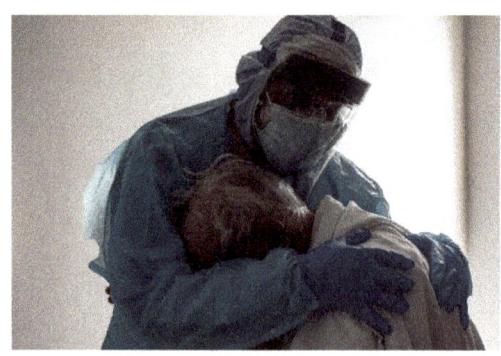

Photo by Go Nakamura/Getty Images 11/26/2020

The above photo posted on Thanksgiving 2020 immediately drove me to tears. It freezes in time to Dr. Joseph Varon in full PPE, comforting an elderly lonely patient in the Covid-ICU in a Houston hospital. The photographer, Go Nakamura, had already visited this ICU twenty times before, attempting to capture what the public does not see- the human toll of such a deadly virus. He managed to also bear witness to human compassion, perhaps the best therapeutic ever.

Dr. Varon had already worked more than 250 days straight. He was fatigued, as were all the other members of the healthcare staff. He was sacrificing his time away from his family on a holiday, placing himself at risk of becoming ill or carrying home the virus to others. I wonder if this hug helped to comfort him, too?

So many people remained resistant to simple public health measures. Some persisted in disbelief, even when sick and dying, that they could possibly have contracted the virus. Was anyone listening to the pleas of healthcare authorities? I watched on TV as large numbers of travelers were seen at the airports, gathering around Thanksgiving tables and in stores doing Black Friday shopping. Really?

"Dark days" were predicted as the number of infected cases increased. We already knew that hospitalizations and deaths would follow in a matter of weeks after holiday gatherings. But the public messaging was all about vaccines that were on the cusp of being prepared to begin distribution, even though there would not be near-term sufficient quantities to protect everyone. Immediate immunity was not guaranteed. People were assuming that things would quickly normalize with our former way of life, but that was a pipe dream. We would still need to wear masks in public in the foreseeable future.

Healthcare workers were still getting sick from Covid. They continued to not have the right kind of quantities of PPE. They were exhausted and burnt out. They were totally frustrated with the mixed messaging from leaders and the lack of concern about getting this pandemic under control. One of my ER colleagues recently said:

"People can't call us heroes, and then go to a BBQ. We are called angels, while they go to a packed church service. Our sacrifices are heralded, but then everyone is clamoring for everything to open up too soon."

Barely out of training, graduates and seasoned veterans were now quitting their jobs, saying, "I'm done. Just done". When asked what they would do instead in an online survey of Emergency Department nurses, 383 comments included switching careers to be a "Walmart Greeter" or "Bus Driver." "Open my own coffee café," "Florist," and so on.

We will eventually see how a shortage of healthcare workers will transform access to care and quality of care. Some locations in the U.S. have already seen this. When the Javits Center in NYC opened as a COVID alternate care site, the ratio of nurses to patients was 1:30.

We all are aware of the long-term effects of disasters. Twenty years ago, 9/11 resulted in many firefighters and first responders becoming ill from the effects of having breathed in toxic fumes and dust. Covid-19 may have long-term effects for a significant number of people as well.

Reports are being assembled about COVID-19 long-haulers who continue to exhibit a myriad of symptoms months after their illness. The potential economic consequences are enormous. It is time to make this personal. Will generations of chronically fatigued people not be able to play with their kids, ride a bike, or work at a job they enjoy because they get too out of breath?

Dr. B. Calinawagan said it best, in my opinion:

"We, the healthcare workers, are not your Frontliners any longer. We are your LAST LINE OF DEFENSE. YOU, my fellow people, are the Frontliners now. The war has shifted to the community, and it is up to you. This cannot be won in the confines of the hospital."

I dreamed of a different photo as the end of 2020 drew near. What if the community firmly rallied around healthcare workers and demonstrated compassion for their service by embracing the personal challenge of being accountable for their own behavior?

The Way Forward   12-9-2020

This past week, there was an exponential increase in COVID-19 cases across the U.S. We are not yet winning this war; we are losing badly.

My brother, Blaise, as predicted, was now the only physician serving his small critical access hospital in rural Wisconsin. The nursing home attached to the hospital currently had a significant outbreak, with 31 out of the 41 residents ill with COVID-19. Deaths were already occurring. Staff were sick as well.

It got so on a past weekend last that the Director of Nursing, who had just returned from her COVID-19 illness, had to work the night shift because there was no one else to work. She was 70 years old. Mask use in the surrounding community remained very spotty.

So, I thought to deeply consider what could be done to ensure that everyone is on the same page in our communities and that the messaging is clear.

Maybe dealing with this pandemic is not unlike other battles to get people to buckle their seatbelts in their vehicles, increase helmet usage, and lower the incidence of alcohol-related tragedies. My prior work as a project coordinator for Safe Communities with the National Highway Traffic Safety Administration gave me some insight into effecting change.

First, we needed a coordinated, multi-pronged approach to change behavior. This approach could be undertaken as the four E's—education, Engineering and Technology, Enforcement, and Economic incentives. If these countermeasures are undertaken concurrently, they are synergistic with each other.

For example, if you want to reduce the number of bike-related head injuries, explain why and how helmets protect our heads; create bike pathways that are separated from roadways; enact state laws to mandate helmet use; and reduce pricing or create insurance incentives for helmet wearers. Visual methods work to demonstrate this.

Education is a foundational element. There have been a lot of "Wear a Mask" signs, yet there are still those who do not understand why they are so critical, wear them reluctantly or only if required where they are going, and may still not wear them correctly.

My niece teaches in-person kindergarten in Boston. Her students all wear their masks diligently the right way. She made sure of it, or they could not attend class. Children can educate their parents. It is logical to think that it should be the other way around; parents should teach their children, and many do. But children can push the case.

An elderly neighbor told me a story about her son wanting to fly down to Florida for a visit. His young daughter began crying and saying that she didn't want her daddy to get sick or to expose grandma and grandpa to the virus. Only because she stood her ground, so adamant about the risk, did he concede to delay traveling. Children can serve as ambassadors for public health in their communities.

It is said that you can reach 95% of the population through the schools. Students, teachers, parents, grandparents, volunteers, janitorial staff, cafeteria personnel, and administrators. We should take advantage of this network.

In disasters, people want to know two things- what is going on, and what do they have to do. We have many in our communities who do not read a newspaper, have an online subscription, or listen to daily news. Social media tends to cover sensational news very superficially and it breeds misinformation and conspiracy theories. We need to clamp down hard on such inaccurate representations of critical information.

I also think we need to talk more about the long-term disability effects of contracting Covid. These are only beginning to be better understood and include multi-system consequences. Some have only been seen when advanced imaging is completed to highlight the cardiac and pulmonary scarring and clots, neurological impacts ranging from headaches to cognitive deficits affecting memory, and an assortment of other issues. One that was discussed this past week was erectile dysfunction in men. Would getting the word out on that type of disability make a difference?

We need to clamp down harder on large public and private gatherings, bars, and clubs. Citations need to be issued even if there can be no monetary cost to them. It needs to be viewed as a criminal occurrence to deliberately be maskless and in crowds at this time.

America needs to manufacture its own PPE. At this time, there is still a shortage of masks, gowns, and even gloves. Healthcare and EMS providers still worry if they will have the supplies needed for their work to protect them. If they become ill or don't feel safe, there will continue to be an exodus of these trained providers.

A current major focus is on the anticipated arrival of the beginning of a vaccination program. There will be a limited rollout supply, so there is time for people to learn about the amazing work behind the development because of advancements in mapping the genomic sequence of COVID.

I do have hope that one day; we can celebrate holidays again, enjoy our families and friends, embrace living in our communities, and travel to faraway places. But we have to do this all together. Everyone. Now.

Pecking Order 1/6/2021

Barnyard animals quickly learn the chain of command among their groups. This is easily evident with chickens. The chicken who pecks the most is considered the alpha chicken, the highest tier.

Unfortunately, there is also a chicken that gets pecked, also known as the Omega one. The other chickens fall somewhere in between.

This concept came to mind as the United States struggles to roll out a mass vaccination campaign. Operation Warp Speed focused on the COVID-19 vaccine development and distribution of the approved product to the states. It was up to the individual states to devise a plan to administer the immunization to residents.

Initially, only the Pfizer vaccine received FDA and CDC approval, and allocations were smaller than expected. Decisions were made to begin vaccinations with healthcare workers, those who faced the greatest risk of being exposed to high viral loads, who provided direct care to persons who became ill from the virus. That made sense to the general public; however, there was a lack of understanding of how big and broad a group this is in the United States.

Even narrowing the initial dosing to direct care providers in the ERs and ICUs of 6,148 hospitals became a major endeavor as it included nurses, doctors, respiratory therapists, environmental services, registration staff, radiology lab personnel, and so on.

The vaccine could not be given to everyone on the same day due to the possibility of side effects that could result in a staff shortage. Even with the now-approved Moderna vaccine allocations, hospitals were *still working* on vaccinating their direct care providers. Then, they still needed to immunize ancillary departmental personnel such as pharmacists, case managers, social workers, central supply staff, etc.

Providing vaccinations for an entire organization was not an easy task. It took dedicated personnel, scheduling, and then detailed documentation into a state database, an immunization card for each person given the injection, and follow-up appointments to ensure the two doses needed for the efficacy of the vaccine. The logistics were much more complex than the annual flu shot campaigns.

The pecking order became visible when hospital staff began posting themselves getting vaccinated. They did this to show their support for the intervention. Hospital administrators also had their photos taken as a show of leadership, even though they were not direct care providers. Rumors trickled related to persons who were vaccinated, who worked mostly remotely, or who did not have inpatient contact.

It did not help to hear that congressional members and their staff were vaccinated in a timely fashion during the initial healthcare rollout. Why do politicians get preference? Would celebrities and athletes also get the first choice?

Another first-tier group to receive vaccinations were residents and staff in long-term care facilities. This was another huge group nationally. Logistics to accomplish this task were even more difficult than hospitals as it required bringing in personnel to administer the shots, scheduling, and care to maintain the critical temperature controls of the drug away from the cold chain storage that many hospitals have. This process was only beginning.

Meantime, private physician providers, home health, fire-rescue, dialysis center staff, oxygen delivery providers and other community healthcare workers were wondering when they will receive their doses.

Community essential workers were further down on the priority list. These included another huge group- those who worked in public safety, communications, transportation, food service, and others. Teachers were being pressured to provide in-person learning, but they were somewhere in the listing, too, with no clue as to when they would receive such protection.

Unfortunately, the public relations nightmare occurred when the CDC and Governors, such as Governor DeSantis in Florida, declared that persons over the age of 65 years should be included in the highest priority group. He held a press conference at a senior residential complex, where 300 vaccine doses were allocated. However, there were 15,000 elders who lived there. There are over 4 million seniors, mostly in the community, living in Florida. They immediately crashed every hotline set up at the hospitals and health department, trying to book an appointment.

Separate allocations were targeted to be distributed to vulnerable populations, including the homeless, those in shelters and prisons, and persons who frequent Federally Qualified Health Centers. There have been questions raised about whether those who are criminals or in the United States illegally should be vaccinated ahead of law-abiding essential workers.

We know that scammers will always try to profit from such an opportunity. Would there be sufficient control over the inevitable black market for vaccines?

The silver lining to all this craziness was that there appeared to be less vaccine hesitancy. Because it was considered a 'scarce resource,' human behavior is such that people crave what is in short supply. There is a sense of entitlement that people demand for themselves what is limited for everyone.

What was desperately needed was more transparency about the logistics needed to get this huge undertaking accomplished. Patience was needed, too. We must all wait for our turn in line. It will happen. Eventually, there will be sufficient supply to vaccinate, hopefully almost everyone, so we can reach the elusive herd immunity level.

The pecking order is one way to maintain control when otherwise it could be a free-for-all. There is much discussion about equitable access to healthcare resources. This is a reality that must be dealt with sensitivity and fairness.

Are we, in the general public, really any better than barnyard animals?

The Hunt   1/22/2021

The pandemic caused a search for scarce resources for everyone. It started early in March of 2020. Reports started trickling in from China, Washington State, and California about a novel coronavirus that was causing outbreaks. There were news clippings of lockdowns abroad and hoarding of items like toilet paper. Toilet paper?

No one anticipated the duration of this disaster. The general thinking was there was a need to hunker down for two weeks only. Then everything magically would go back to normal.

When there is a perception that certain items might become limited, the instinct most people have is to run out and purchase those specific supplies. If their go-to store did not have stock, the hunt began to locate necessities elsewhere.

With the convenience of neighborhood stores, our society has evolved to just-in-time purchasing versus maintaining a supply of staples in our pantries. Even in Florida, where hurricane preparedness for 72 hours is an annual tradition, this did not translate to being year-round prepared for a disaster such as Covid-19.

Social media sites started sharing shopper's personal experiences of finding totally bare shelves in the paper products and cleaning supplies aisles. People were clearly hoarding and the visuals on television escalated such behavior.

How much toilet paper is needed for an average household? It became a comical point that even wound up on Christmas ornaments. But it wasn't just toilet paper.

During the period when there were extensive lockdowns, grocery store shelves started looking barer with gaps apparent on shelves where favorite brands of things had a long-standing place.

People realized that they needed to start cooking their own meals at home regularly instead of relying on going out to restaurants or getting takeout. The pursuit of precious food basics became a priority. Sweet and savory comfort food snacks were also on everyone's grocery list.

The positive part of this was that home baking was resurrected. A bread machine was a hot appliance as long as you could find one and then locate flour and yeast. The usual abundance of fresh vegetables dwindled as many rediscovered meal preparations such as casseroles and soups. A healthy head of lettuce was challenging to find, so salads were not an easy option.

Our hunt for food basics extended to the internet, and we learned to order from Amazon when it was available. Many stores offered curbside pickup or home deliveries, too. We all searched for what we needed, scrolling through virtual shelves and considering substitutions. Would we eventually return to in-store shopping to the degree that we used to?

Things feel a bit more stable now, ten months into this pandemic. We have gotten more creative in finding substitutes for items and are exploring a range of sites to purchase from. But we have a new quest—hunting for a vaccine appointment.

It has been a frustrating experience as demand has far exceeded available supply. It has become another virtual experience, and we are suffering through phone lines that no one answers and multiple online registration portals that crash.

It is just assumed that people will be able to navigate through complex processes that require internet access or a smartphone. Without these technologies, there are many left behind who are losing hope. I feel terrible for those who are in their 90s and are left to beg for help.

I am computer literate and do own an iPhone. However, this has not helped me to be able to succeed on accessing an appointment. Again, this morning, I arose at 5:30 am to logon to our Publix supermarket website, designated as a distribution site in Florida. Even though the alarm was set, I kept waking up during the night again and again to check on the time. I felt stressed and exhausted by the anticipation of it all.

6:00 am arrived, and after a long delay, which appeared that the site had frozen. I saw a popup that said,

Schedule an Appointment

Hooray! I entered basic demographic information (name, address, phone number, gender, birth date). All of that was okay. But then, there were a whole slew of other questions.

Was I a Florida resident? Yes, I was happy to click on that as so many vaccine tourists, over 39,000, were consuming our available shots.

The question-and-answer process was tedious, but I persisted. The screen kept freezing up and then taking me back to the prior page of questions. The site refreshed itself every minute, which slowed everything down.

I got up to the consent part and then was faced with the next challenge. Okay.

I am not a Robot.

I understand why they have this statement, but time was of the essence. So, I plodded through the maze of "Pick all the squares with traffic lights," "Choose all the squares with mountains," "Locate all the bicycles," and "Find all the squares with buses". Come on!

Finally, the program figured out that I was really a human, and took me to:

Continue

Yea! Now I was finally up to the "Schedule an appointment section." But there were more hurdles. In their infinite wisdom, Publix's portal included store vaccination sites in multiple states. I chose Florida and it was no surprise that it froze again for at least 20 minutes. Then, when it became live again, I had to choose a County from the drop –down menu. Frozen again. Finally, it unfroze, and I hit my county. Frozen again.

I waited another 20 minutes for it to unfreeze so I could press Continue.

Yes! The next instruction was:

Choose a Location

No problem. I clicked on the site closest to me, about 12 miles away, but that was fine.

Choose a Time

That was a bit of a surprise as the only available times were from 8 pm on. I clicked the next available time at 8 pm and clicked Continue again. There was a message:

The location and time you chose is no longer available, as the spot has been filled by another customer. Please choose another appointment.

Oh no! It took me way back to the question and answer and Robot page. I did it all again, and again, and again. Three more times with different locations and times. Then, the site issued a final message:

Fully Booked

I gave up for the day and focused on more productive household tasks instead.

Update: An email came through from our Health Department that I could schedule an appointment for the next day! We'll see how this next part of my hunt goes....

Breaking Point 8/15/21

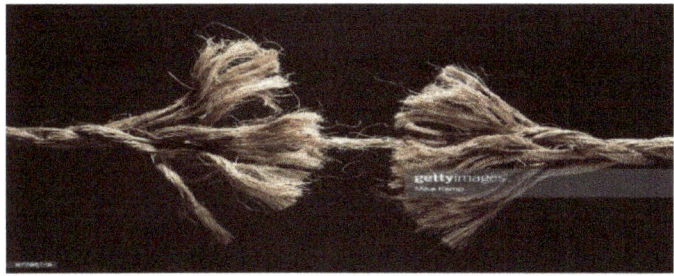

A survey of 188 hospitals in Florida this past week revealed that 68% anticipated a critical staff shortage (doctors, respiratory therapists, and especially nurses) within the next 5-7 days. This is significant as hospitalizations from the Covid Delta variant are on an exponential trajectory.

ER waiting rooms in Florida, and a growing number of other states were filled with ill people waiting to get treated. Some of the wait times have been as long as twelve hours. Those who were deemed as non-immediately life threatened were being directed to Urgent Care Centers instead, but those facilities were over capacity, too.

Seven percent of hospitals were on diversion, meaning they would not accept ambulance-transported patients. It wasn't all COVID-related- the usual car crashes, strokes, heart attacks, and other emergencies still happened. There was no guarantee to be seen and treated quickly by anyone. Delays were just unavoidable with the current conditions.

Admitted patients waited in emergency departments for ICU beds to become available. Sometimes, their wait went on for days. The care received in an overcrowded emergency department is not the same as the care a critical care patient deserves.

Resources were spread too thin. Concerns about oxygen deliveries, medical supplies, and pharmaceuticals continued. Ventilators were limited. There were empty beds in shuttered wards but insufficient staff to care for patients.

Nurses were leaving the bedside as part of an exodus just as this next covid wave was surging. Why?

Healthcare staff shortages were nothing new, and nursing had been particularly affected throughout the profession's history. Insufficient pay and difficult working conditions were previously cited. So, what was different now?

It has been 18 months since the pandemic began in the U.S. Nurses are tired and burnt out. They have been perpetually afraid to bring the virus home to their families. Taking all precautions, stripping in the garage, throwing their contaminated scrubs into the washer, and then immediately showering, praying that no viral particles would remain. Some have slept in their basements or in hotel rooms with colleagues who had the same fear of contaminating others. The fear at work was intense during insufficient and poor-quality PPE supplies. Would they get sick wearing the same mask over and over?

During the first and second pandemic waves, hospital staff rallied and sacrificed, working longer hours in high-stress situations. The communities around hospitals rallied to honor their 'heroes'. Children sent crayon drawings thanking staff for their service. These were proudly displayed on walls in the nurses' lounges, but now they look old and tattered.

The newest wave felt different. Patient ratios were insane, verbal and physical assaults occurred too frequently, documentation expectations remained excessive, and administration was focused on staff recruitment instead of on what would support the retention of loyal personnel. So, staff have left the hospital workforce. Many nurses took travel positions with more generous pay, went to other types of jobs, or just decided to retire early.

There was now prevalent compassion fatigue, frustration, and anger that may not have been visible externally, but it was there. Instead, it was becoming evident in social media posts. Being unvaccinated and ill was now viewed as a predictable, preventable tragedy harming those around the infected. Some have compared it to thousands of drunk drivers who can hurt themselves and any innocents in their way when they crash. No one wants to shame those who are hesitant, resistant to getting vaccinated, or are already ill. Still, a palpable undercurrent exists that such persons are contributing to the variant strains.

Staff have exceeded their physical, mental, and moral limits. The 'heroes' are now tired and broken. They have been their patients' lifelines to their families, holding iPads up so those needing intubation or approaching the end of their lives could say goodbye to their loved ones. Despite strenuous efforts to save them, patients were dying in multiples within the ERs, ICUs, the floors, and at home. Walking past the refrigerated morgue trucks outside the hospital was a sobering reality check.

The Delta variant hit people hard and could be quickly overwhelming. This time around, there were children who were becoming ill, too. There were too few Children's Hospitals or Pediatric beds available. Many hospitals no longer even had a pediatric service.

Nurses became sick as they were exposed to the highest viral loads. In the first 12 months of the pandemic in 2020, 3600 nurses died. It would not be surprising if the number exceeded 5,000 during 2021. Unfortunately, there were still too many unvaccinated healthcare workers- less than 50%. One of my ER colleagues wound up admitted to an ICU with bilateral pneumonia. He had required a ventilator for over 10 days. Now, he has blood clots in his legs and needs dialysis. It is unclear if he will survive. He was unvaccinated. His recovery, if he makes it, will be a long one. Another bedside nurse is gone. (Sadly, he did die.)

Statements from nurses have included.

"I don't have any strength left. Honestly, I've given so much I can't keep going. It's affected me in ways I never thought possible. It's not getting better, and I have to protect myself and my family and my sanity."

"There was never a time that we could just kind of take a breath. I hit that point... I can't do this anymore. I'm just so tapped out."

"Today I worked with teammates for 45 minutes doing compressions to save a coworker. The tears didn't really flow until I sat in my car when I could decompress."

My time working clinically is over. I still get dozens of daily emails from hospitals and agencies looking for ER nurses in every state. Some offer as much as a $20,000 bonus to work for two years. Even though I know things are at a breaking point and healthcare systems are in danger of collapsing, this is a situation that will need a major strategy to correct. Healthcare can no longer be run as a business with profits made on the backs of staff. It is time to fix this.

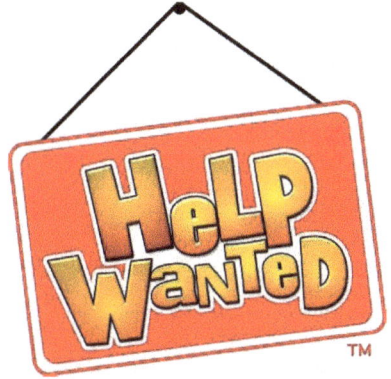

Are we there yet?   11/3/2021

It is now 18 months that we have been dealing with this Covid-19 pandemic. Everyone is tired of it. It doesn't seem to matter what age you are. We have all been impacted. It reminds me of young children on a long car ride who keep asking "Are we there yet?"

What impressions have I gathered from people I know? In my large extended family, I try to rotate, catching up with each person as I can. Some are good communicators, and others do not reciprocate when picking up the phone to call. It's always been like that, I suppose, but it still surprises me during these years of crisis that the non-communicators do not reach out a bit more. Without family gatherings, like birthday parties, weddings, reunions, or even funerals, we may have grown distant from each other's lives more than in normal times.

Many of us continue in our bubbles of existence, being cautious about higher density crowds and travel. Even though my husband and I are fully vaccinated, even with a booster, we still worry about the mutant viral covid strains, most recently now the mu strain.

There are still outbreaks erupting in some states like Alaska, Colorado, Maine, New Hampshire and New Mexico, in which hospital admissions increased 15% in the last two weeks. It's no surprise as vaccinations rates nationally are only at 58%, so we are nowhere near herd immunity. Alaska's outbreak is so severe that pregnant women are being told that if they go into labor, they should plan on delivering their babies at home!

It depends on where you live and the degree of restrictions there are. At our summer residence in Nantucket, Massachusetts, public health measures are clearly communicated and enforced. In South Florida, where we spend our winters, it is the total opposite. Masks are required for healthcare visits, including our local pharmacy, but elsewhere, there is mass non-compliance.

It is impossible to know who has gotten their COVID shots or not. We know that most of the kids under 12 years old have not yet been vaccinated. It will be interesting to see if their parents and pediatricians can encourage such a protective measure.

What child would willingly want an injection? And two shots? The possibility of having to get a shot at my annual physical when I was young was extremely anxiety-producing. I saw the same concern when my own children were small.

I anticipate that we will have to wear masks intermittently even when this whole COVID virus diminishes. I fear that there will be another virus to take its place. Will we ever be able to see each other smile again, or talk freely without a face covering? How many people will get a flu shot this year? A bad flu season or a "twindemic" of both COVID and flu infections could be devastating.

People demonstrate how they feel in different ways. Some insist on traveling, regardless of the risks and delays associated with air travel and Uber/Lyft transportation these days. When my husband and I took our return trip to Florida, I was shocked at how many young people, especially, were traveling. Maybe the cheaper bargain flights or the fact that they are either not working or working remotely allows them the flexibility to fly the coop.

People are booking again on cruises. Several brothers and sisters have plans for fall and winter destinations. How can they feel safe among two thousand or more other people?

2021 is being called the year of "The Great Resignation." Many feel dissatisfied with their current employment. People say they want a higher salary, better benefits, and management that cares about them. Working remotely brought a life-work balance that is not easy to give up and return to an in-person office routine. The end result is "Now Hiring" signs in the windows of restaurants and businesses.

The supply chain is still being greatly affected. Container ships are lined up waiting to be unloaded, but that will require 24/7 dock workers. In addition, there is a shortage of truck drivers to transport goods to stores and businesses. It is still hit or miss at the grocery store for what is available, although it has improved somewhat. You just can't plan on always getting the brand you want. The quality of items like paper goods has also been affected. Parents have concerns about being able to locate their favorite toys for the upcoming holidays, so there is a big push to get the supply chain functioning again.

The level of anger, frustration, and violence has increased everywhere. I worry about further escalation, especially because political viewpoints are so divisive. Law enforcement is struggling to hire new officers due to public perceptions. I am closely watching the vote for the Minneapolis Police Department to be completely disbanded.

My heart still worries about my healthcare colleagues facing an unrelenting stream of people needing care. It's not just COVID anymore. It is also people who put off checkups or have chronic conditions that just got worse. Staffing shortages are rampant. Hospital beds may exist, but without personnel to staff them. The turnover rate is unsurpassed, and staff who remain loyal to feel even more stressed as they have to train new hires and supervise some very inexperienced people. Those who can retire do so.

Anyone who teaches can share stories of these difficult times. There is a prevalent lack of energy and ambition on the part of both students and those providing instruction.

One of my nieces is a first-year kindergarten teacher in a public elementary school. She was a substitute teacher for a semester, but with the lack of enough other experienced educators, she was put in charge of her own class this year. She is supposed to only have 17 students in her class. Instead, there are 22, 4 of whom do not speak any English. She never took any education classes in college nor received formal training from her school district.

Another of my nieces also teaches at an elementary school in Staten Island. She has years of training and experience but is also very stressed. The mask mandates were a source of regular concern. What is so hard about wearing a mask correctly? The irony is that as soon as class is dismissed for the day, the masks come off, and the students congregate together outdoors.

School boards have been in the news, with contentious parents speaking out about the COVID restrictions, quarantining policy, mask mandates, and so on.

My son teaches at a university level, and he sounds tired. Student attendance is spotty; assignments are not always as good as they should be and turned in on time. However, the challenges for students are real, too. He has had students in the hospital for COVID-19 and students who have lost family members. Everyone is in survival mode, trying to slog through the semester.

So, are we there yet? No. The last major pandemic took two full years, and this one looks like it will also last as long. I am hopeful that we will eventually reach a new normal though. Hopefully, we will all remember what we did to keep ourselves safe during this pandemic. Or pass on those lessons learned for future generations.

Bubble Town   1/5/22

"My toddler doesn't know what 'normal' is. She is now two years old and only knows what living in a bubble is like. Her world is so small". This comment was made by my niece during a Christmas Eve phone conversation.

It used to be that we were worried about crime on our streets. Now, it's a totally different thing. The predators we are most fearful of are the Covid variants, the most recent of which is Omicron.

When the Alpha variant arrived in early 2020, it did scare us into lockdowns, school closures, and remote working. Most of us had never heard of a coronavirus and spike proteins. Few knew how to correctly wear a mask.

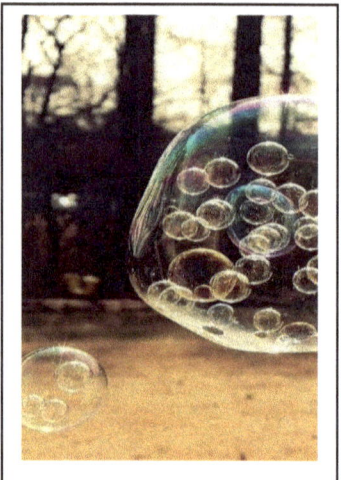

It was the first time that the phrase "living in a bubble" surfaced. We canceled travel plans, had quarantine birthdays, delivered food and supplies to our homes, and hunkered down. Our favorite pastime became watching Netflix movies. When we did venture out of our bubbles, we had to constantly remind ourselves to bring masks with us. We began keeping extras in our cars and pockets. We were individual bubbles outside of our bubble homes.

Those of us who lived in bubbles, bubble people, only trusted each other and preferred to associate with like-minded people who carefully followed the rules. Our bubbles coalesced with others and collectively formed a Bubble Town.

Unfortunately, the elderly in nursing homes and those who lived in high-density housing became vulnerable to the virus. People were getting sick, but it seemed like it was mostly in urban areas or those who provided essential services in their communities.

The virus was insidious, though, and sought out those who were resistant to following public health guidance, especially those who did not or could not live in a bubble.

When the vaccine became available beginning at the end of 2020, the supplies and rollout took time to implement through 2021. We all thought that being double vaccinated was going to free us from the pandemic. The summer of 2021 looked hopeful, and people were excited to travel again and enjoy outdoor dining. The momentum picked up, and it seemed like there was no going back to being confined again. Mask-wearing diminished, and most of us became complacent.

The vaccines demonstrated that they did make a difference when the Delta variant emerged in 2021 and afflicted mostly unvaccinated young and middle-aged adults. Getting 'boosted' for waning immunity among those vaccinated became a new priority in the fall of 2021.

The influence of politics and social media disinformation played a significant role in not achieving the goal of 'herd immunity.' We began blaming those who were hesitant or resistant to getting immunized. Our hospital capacities remained stretched, with full ERs and ICUs.

This newest incredibly transmissible mutated virus, Omicron, is hitting many of us all at once now in early 2022 at an exponential rate. It seeks out vulnerable hosts among those still unvaccinated and even those vaccinated and boosted. It is particularly problematic that children under five years of age are becoming ill, and pediatric hospitalizations have increased dramatically within the last two weeks. It is anticipated to become much worse.

Omicron has grabbed our attention because so many of us are now sick. Call-outs of essential workers, already working with staff shortages, are now exacerbated. To make matters worse, influenza is also rearing its ugly head too. The predominant strain is not included in this year's flu vaccine.

We are being driven back into living within bubbles. When venturing out, we are again wearing masks and keeping our distance from others who may be infected.

There are still people who refuse to be part of mitigating infectious diseases. Instead of choosing to be in a protective bubble, they collectively stew in their own petri dishes within cruise ships, holiday parties, football games, and concerts. It seems like there is no reasoning with such stalwart people.

The cruise industry is big in South Florida. People fly in from all over the U.S. to enjoy the sunny destinations in the Caribbean or Bahamas. The cruise lines insist that they are following all CDC protocols, so passengers will be safe from the virus. Like they are in their own protective bubble. Not so.

In the past week, ninety cruise ships had COVID outbreaks, with more than 5,000 passengers infected. The cruise ships had to either return to port or stay offshore for a week, and most were denied access to island trips.

Unfortunately, when outbreaks occur, the bubbles burst, and those inside the afflicted bubbles fall out. It is fascinating that people assume that if they get COVID, they will be quickly treated at hospitals and receive monoclonal antibodies or witch-doctor remedies like Ivermectin or 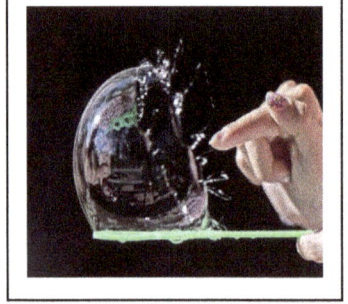 hydroxychloroquine. Two of the three monoclonal antibody medications are not effective against Omicron, and the remaining one is in short supply. There are those who falsely believe that if they became ill, then they could choose to be vaccinated. For many, it will be too late.

If hospitalized with COVID, people will be shocked that they will be placed in bubble jail- isolation. A family member might be allowed if they are dying. Otherwise, they are completely alone.

Their caretakers, nurses, and doctors will also be outfitted with bubble protective suits. Their faces will be barely visible through the layers of plastic and masks.

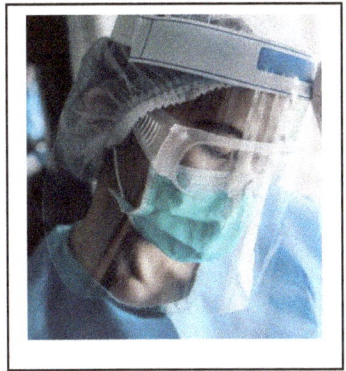

There continues to be an exodus among hospital and nursing home staff leaving their jobs. They cite burnout, moral injury, and the stress of always working short-staffed. Elective surgeries are cancelled again, visitor restrictions are in place, and those needing admission are being held waiting in ERs for many hours or days. The strain on the healthcare system is overwhelming. What does all of this mean for the future? We will need to live with a constant threat of emerging infectious diseases. Protective measures such as mask wearing need to remain in place for all mass transportation and public settings, such as government and within healthcare facilities. There has to be accountability for misinformation and refusal to abide by community health practices. Otherwise, the future may look like this.

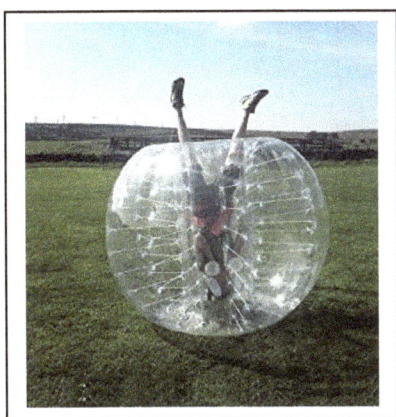
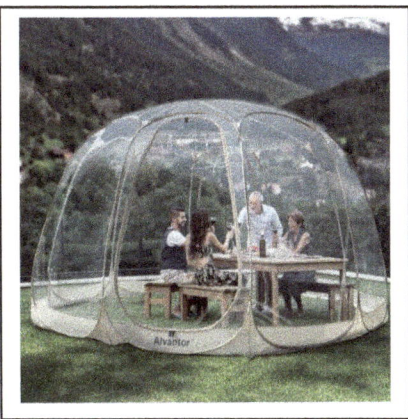

ACKNOWLEDGMENTS

I have worked with amazing people throughout my life. Taking good care of people takes a team. On night shifts especially, we bonded because we were in terms of staffing to deal with whatever hit our doorstep. Boca Raton Regional Hospital (now Baptist Health) was an incredible place to work, and I am grateful for its dedicated doctors, paramedics, administrative staff, and nurses. For those who have worked with me and recall some of these stories, you know who you are, and I am thankful that you were there with me.

Much of what we saw regarding illnesses or injuries was routine and predictable. It was amazing that people can still come up with novel problems and mechanisms of injury. The stories I have told in this book are just some of them. You have to maintain humility, as you have never seen it all, and emotions can run strong in some instances.

Nursing involves lifelong learning, and it can feel consuming to stay current with technology, new medications, treatment protocols, and policies. I found that my professional memberships in Critical Care (AACN)and Emergency Nursing (ENA) were helpful for staying current. Joining committees and accepting presentation invitations connected me to a vast network of colleagues. I never felt alone.

Writing these stories was cathartic. I need to recognize my Nantucket Writing Group for being a safe space to talk about and write down my experiences. I could tell that sometimes the stories were shocking as none of them 'lived' in my world of being a nurse. I could also tell that they felt the deep emotions that I tried to get down on paper.

I am grateful to my husband, Don, and my two children, David and Karen, who kept me grounded over the years. My soul mate, Susan, whom I met through her family tragedy and tirelessly joined me with community injury prevention activities, has read every one of my stories and commented on them.

My Graduate School of Nursing classmates have remained in touch through a yearly newsletter, and we have shared life's passages together in addition to our careers.

There was a lot more to my career that I have not written about in terms of disaster work and public health. Perhaps another set of stories one day.

ABOUT THE AUTHOR

Mary Russell grew up in New York and graduated from Russell Sage College in Troy, New York, with a B.S. in Physical Therapy. She then enrolled in Pace University's Graduate School of Nursing to earn an MSN. She has worked in rehabilitation, Critical Care Units, Burn Units, Emergency Departments, Community Health, and Public Health.

She earned her Doctorate in Education from Florida International University as part of her goal to support public education in injury prevention. She served as the Director of the Safe Communities program at Florida Atlantic University, and she was appointed a faculty appointment in the College of Nursing.

She has authored publications on motor vehicle injury prevention, hospital emergency management, and other topics.

Currently, she supports the development of emergency preparedness resources as a Subject Matter Expert for the U.S. Department of Health and Human Services, Administration for Strategic Preparedness and Response (ASPR) Technical Research, Assistance Center and Information Exchange (TRACIE). She also continues to serve on the Healthcare Emergency Response Coalition of Palm Beach County, Florida.

www.ingramcontent.com/pod-product-compliance
Lightning Source LLC
Chambersburg PA
CBHW051521120626

46551CB00012B/1020